N SITE

CASE HISTORIES FOR THE MRCP

'Fully updated in line with new MRCP exam format'

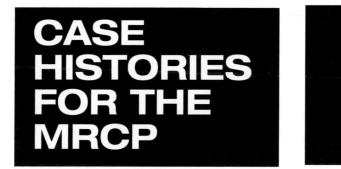

CASE HISTORIES FOR THE MRCP

Second edition

Paul Goldsmith MA BM BCh PhD MRCP

Specialist Registrar in Neurology,
Addenbrooke's Hospital, Cambridge, UK

Robert Semple MA MB BChir MRCP(UK)

Wellcome Trust Clinical Research Training
Fellow in Diabetes and Endocrinology,
Addenbrooke's Hospital, Cambridge, UK

ARNOLD

A member of the Hodder Headline Group
LONDON

First published in Great Britain in 2004 by
Arnold, a member of the Hodder Headline Group,
338 Euston Road, London NW1 3BH

http://www.arnoldpublishers.com

Distributed in the United States of America by
Oxford University Press Inc.,
198 Madison Avenue, New York, NY10016
Oxford is a registered trademark of Oxford University Press

Whilst the advice and information in this book are believed to be true and
accurate at the date of going to press, neither the authors nor the publisher
can accept any legal responsibility or liability for any errors or omissions
that may be made. In particular (but without limiting the generality of the
preceding disclaimer) every effort has been made to check drug dosages;
however, it is still possible that errors have been missed. Furthermore,
dosage schedules are constantly being revised and new side-effects
recognized. For these reasons the reader is strongly urged to consult the
drug companies' printed instructions before administering any of the drugs
recommended in this book.

British Library Cataloguing in Publication Data
A catalogue record for this book is available from the British Library

Library of Congress Cataloging-in-Publication Data
A catalog record for this book is available from the Library of Congress

ISBN 0 340 81037 8

1 2 3 4 5 6 7 8 9 10

Commissioning Editor: Joanna Koster
Project Editor: Wendy Rooke
Production Controller: Deborah Smith
Cover Design: Amina Dudhia

Typeset in 10/12 Sabon by Charon Tec. Pvt. Ltd, Chennai
Printed and bound in Italy

What do you think about this book? Or any other Arnold title?
Please send your comments to **feedback.arnold@hodder.co.uk**

Contents

Answers

Acknowledgements

Medicine is a lifelong apprenticeship. We have both been fortunate to work with many skilled and perspicacious clinicians, from whom we have learned much, and continue to learn. The observations in this book are largely based on real cases. We thank our teachers for our own education.

We would like to thank a number of individuals who have kindly allowed us to reproduce their illustrations in this book:

Dr B.R. Allen, Mr J. Anderson, Mr J. Bancewicz, Dr D.H. Bennett, Professor Sir N.L. Browse, Dr A.Y. Butt, Professor P.A. Corris, Professor R.E. Cotton, Dr J. Curtis, Dr F. Dudley Hart, Professor H. Ellis, Dr C.C. Evans, Professor S. Field, Professor R.G. Finch, Dr D. Gray, Professor T.W. Higenbottam, Dr I.D.A. Johnston, Dr J.T. Macfarlane, Dr A.M. McLean, Professor R. Marks, Professor N.J. Mortensen, Mr J. Murie, Dr W.L. Nyhan, Dr C.M. Ogilvie, Dr S.T.D. Roxburgh, Mr R.C.G. Russell, Dr R.C.D. Staughton, Dr J. Stevens, Dr P.J. Toghill, Professor T. Treasure, Professor G.H. Whitehouse, Dr L.A. Wilson

Additional illustration acknowledgements:

Illustrations appearing in Case 6.1 and Case 14.10 reproduced with permission from Taylor, D. & Hoyt, C., *Practical Paediatric Ophthalmology*; published by Blackwell Science, 1997

Illustration appearing in Case 20.5 reproduced from Durrington, P.N., *Hyperlipidaemia*, second edition; Butterworth Heinemann, 1995. Original source: Holt, L.E. *et al*, Idiopathic familial lipaemia. *Johns Hopkins Hospital Bulletin*, **64**, 279–314 (1939)

Introduction

The dramatic changes in medical training over the past six years have included an overhaul of the MRCP examinations. To address this, *Case Histories for the MRCP* has been completely rewritten to mirror the style of the new examination and thus to optimize the preparation of the prospective candidate. Some cases have been removed and new ones have been added. Many are now integrated cases involving case history, data handling and picture interpretation. Answers are in the new 'select from a range of possibilities' style. While the format has changed, two integral features of the first edition have been maintained. First, we make no apologies that these questions are tough: easy questions provide false reassurance. We aim to help give candidates the edge in those difficult questions that discriminate at the top end of the field. Second, we have retained in-depth explanations of why we think the given answer to be best, as engagement in the process of clinical reasoning is not only a key aim of the book but also, we believe, the best way to acquire the skills that are tested in the MRCP examination.

Robert Semple has joined me as co-author for this second edition. His extensive MRCP teaching experience and ongoing general medicine training as a medical specialist registrar at Addenbrooke's Hospital have helped ensure the value and relevance of this book.

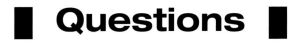

Questions

Exam 1

█████████

Case 1.1

A 66-year-old retired sheep farmer presents with a persistent cough, dating from a cold some nine months ago. He has become more short of breath on exercise, and he wheezes occasionally, although he dismisses these symptoms as being due to his increasing weight following retirement. On examination, he is short, stocky and overweight. His breathing is somewhat noisy but his chest is clear on auscultation. Neurological examination is normal. There is no fatigability.

Full blood count and electrolytes are normal. ESR 7 mm/h. Static and dynamic lung volumes are normal (FEV_1 2.8 l). PEFR 200 l/min.

1. Which of the following pathologies best fits this clinical scenario?
   a) Hypersensitivity pneumonitis
   b) Chronic obstructive pulmonary disease
   c) Obstructive sleep apnoea
   d) Multinodular goitre

2. Choose the three initial investigations most likely to be helpful:
   a) Plain chest radiograph
   b) Flow-volume loop
   c) Serum precipitins
   d) Serum IgE
   e) Serial peak flows
   f) CT chest/neck
   g) Bronchoscopy
   h) Polysomnography

Case 1.2

A 22-year-old student presented with a three-day history of a severe sore throat. During the previous 24 hours he had developed a tender neck, rigors, increasing shortness of breath, and a cough productive of purulent sputum. There was no past medical history, infectious contacts, foreign travel or intravenous drug abuse. On examination he was extremely unwell.

Temperature 39.8 °C. Blood pressure 100/50 mmHg. Pulse 120 bpm.

He had marked pharyngitis and tender cervical lymphadenopathy. His respiratory rate was 30/min and diffuse chest crepitations were audible. The chest radiograph is shown below:

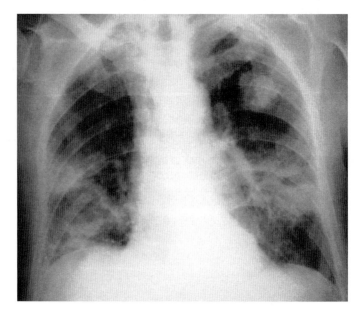

Ultrasound of the neck showed a non-compressible right internal jugular vein with no detectable blood flow.

1. Choose the single best diagnosis from the following:
    a) Infectious mononucleosis
    b) Vincent's angina
    c) Group A streptococcal infection
    d) Lemierre's disease
    e) Lymphoreticular malignancy

2. Which of the following treatments would you institute?
    a) Supportive care only
    b) Intravenous benzylpenicillin and metronidazole
    c) Intravenous benzylpenicillin
    d) Intravenous aciclovir, ciprofloxacin and fluconazole
    e) High-dose oral phenoxymethylpenicillin

Case 1.3

A 56-year-old lady presented with a month's history of intermittent high fevers. Her only past medical history was of type 2 diabetes controlled by tolbutamide. There were no other symptoms or features of note in the history. Specifically, she had never been abroad or exposed to TB and she had no animal exposure. On examination, she was febrile at 38.2 °C, but no other abnormality was detected.

Hb 10.2 g/dl. White cell count $8.3 \times 10^9/l$. Rheumatoid factor, ANA and AMA all negative. Syphilis, hepatitis A, B and C, HIV, *Toxoplasma*, *Brucella*, CMV, EBV and *Toxocara* serology all negative. Complement levels normal. CT abdomen and thorax normal. Repeated blood cultures and urine culture negative. Serial early morning urine samples negative for AFBs. Tuberculin testing (to one in 10) negative.

Liver function tests were abnormal, however, prompting a liver biopsy, which showed non-caseating granulomata. No bacilli were seen with the Warthin–Starry stain. Silver staining and specific immunostaining were normal. The bile ducts were preserved. There was no response to an empirical course of anti-tuberculous chemotherapy.

1. Choose the most appropriate next step from the following:
   a) Bronchoalveolar lavage and biopsy
   b) Indium-labelled white cell scintigraphy
   c) Colonoscopy and biopsy
   d) Kveim test
   e) Analysis of T-cell receptor gene rearrangements
   f) Withdrawal of tolbutamide
   g) *Bartonella* serology
   h) Course of corticosteroids
   i) PCR of liver tissue for *Tropheryma whippelii*

2. Should the first step fail to suggest a diagnosis, choose a further course of action from the above list.

Case 1.4

A 30-year-old lady presented with increasing shortness of breath over six months. An echocardiogram supported the clinical diagnosis of a dilated cardiomyopathy. Angiography excluded an ischaemic cause. Her past medical history was unremarkable, although she had gone through the menopause prematurely two years previously. She deteriorated rapidly, and underwent an emergency cardiac transplant. The surgeon made the diagnosis.

1. Which of the following additional findings would be consistent with the unifying diagnosis?
   a) Bitemporal hemianopia
   b) History of postpartum haemorrhage

c) Erythema nodosum
d) Strongly positive thyroid autoantibodies
e) Radiographic evidence of chondrocalcinosis

Case 1.5

A 45-year-old man presented with a four-month history of episodic dizziness pro-voked by sudden head movement together with a lack of co-ordination. In his past medical history, he had had an atrial septal defect (ASD) corrected surgically at age 12. More recently he had been taking sleeping tablets following the death of his mother from a renal cell carcinoma. On examination, he exhibited rotatory nystagmus on left gaze, cerebellar signs in his left arm, and an ataxic gait veering to the left. Cranial nerve and limb examination was otherwise normal.

1. Select the best diagnosis from the following:
    a) Left-sided cerebellar haemangioblastoma
    b) Right-sided cerebellar haemangioblastoma
    c) Left-sided cerebellar signs secondary to sleeping tablet toxicity
    d) Right-sided cerebellar signs secondary to sleeping tablet toxicity
    e) Left-sided cerebellar medulloblastoma
    f) Right-sided cerebellar medulloblastoma
    g) Lowes syndrome (oculo-cerebro-renal syndrome)

2. Choose the single most pertinent investigation from each of the following three groups:
    a) MRI posterior fossa
    b) Sleeping tablet toxicity screen
    c) Renal biopsy

    d) Haemoglobin estimation
    e) Creatinine levels
    f) Creatine levels
    g) Caeruloplasmin levels

    h) Retinal angiography
    i) Slit-lamp examination of cornea
    j) Slit-lamp examination of lens
    k) Oculonystagmography

Case 1.6

A 58-year-old builder presented with an eight-hour history of left iliac fossa pain. He felt nauseated and he had vomited once. While waiting for the ambulance he had a bout of diarrhoea, in which he thought he could see blood. He had suffered with similar, but milder, pain over the preceding two months, which he thought was associated with food. In his past medical history, he had well-controlled angina for four years and grade 1 sarcoidosis at age 25, which settled spontaneously. On examination, his temperature was 37.8 °C. His left iliac fossa was tender, although there was no guarding. Bowel sounds were present and rectal examination was normal. No other abnormality was detected.

A plain abdominal radiograph of the patient is shown below:

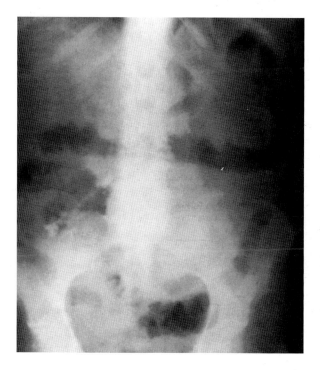

1. Which of the following best describes this appearance?
   a) Rigler's sign is positive
   b) It is within normal limits
   c) There is evidence of toxic megacolon
   d) There is evidence of colonic mucosal oedema
   e) It shows a 'drainpipe' colon

2. What is the most likely diagnosis?
   a) Inflammatory bowel disease
   b) Sigmoid diverticulosis
   c) Ischaemic colitis
   d) Colonic carcinoma
   e) Colonic infarction

3. What is the next investigation?
   a) Rigid sigmoidoscopy and biopsy
   b) Double-contrast barium enema
   c) Mesenteric angiography
   d) Exploratory laparotomy
   e) Colonoscopy and biopsy

Case 1.7

An 18-year-old carpenter presented with pain in his right loin. Two months previously he had passed some grit in his urine. His GP had sent a sample of urine for microscopy. This reported the presence of hexagonal crystals. His past medical history was otherwise unremarkable, and he took no medications. His uncle had a history of renal stones. Examination was normal except for a tender right flank.

Hb 13.5 g/dl, white cell count $14.6 \times 10^9/l$. Electrolytes, liver function, calcium and phosphate all normal. 24-hour urine calcium excretion normal. Intravenous pyelogram (IVP) faintly radio-opaque stag-horn calculus in right renal pelvis. No evidence of collecting system cysts.

1. What is the diagnosis?
   a) Chronic *Proteus* infection complicated by magnesium ammonium phosphate calculus
   b) Cystinosis
   c) Type 1 hyperoxaluria
   d) Cystinuria
   e) Type 2 hyperoxaluria

2. Choose one confirmatory investigation from the following:
   a) Urine sodium nitroprusside test
   b) Serial midstream urine samples for culture, and culture of stones
   c) Ehrlich's aldehyde test of urine
   d) Urinary oxalate assay
   e) Urinary citrate assay

Case 1.8

A 78-year-old lady was found collapsed in her bedroom at her residential home. She had got up to go to the toilet and discovered a weakness on one side of her body. Her past medical history was unremarkable except for bad osteoarthritis of her knees and hips. She smoked ten cigarettes per day and enjoyed her sherry. She took ibuprofen for pain. On examination, she had a right homonymous hemianopia and right-sided facial weakness. She had an expressive dysphasia. The remainder of the cranial nerve examination was normal. In her limbs she had grade 3/5 weakness on the right in a pyramidal distribution, with corresponding hyperreflexia and an up-going right plantar. Her blood pressure was 170/95 mmHg and a left carotid bruit was audible. The remainder of the examination was normal.

Hb 12.5 g/dl, white cell count 12.4 × 10^9/l (neutrophils 70%, lymphocytes 29%), platelets 330 × 10^9/l, clotting studies normal, Na 138 mmol/l, K 5.4 mmol/l, urea 28.5 mmol/l, creatinine 550 μmol/l, albumin 38 g/l, Ca 1.7 mmol/l, PO_4 2.2 mmol/l, urate 480 μmol/l (normal: 150–390 μmol/l). CXR and ECG normal.

1. What is the likely cause of the renal failure?
    a) Rhabdomyolysis
    b) Hypertension
    c) NSAID-induced damage
    d) Hypoparathyroidism

2. Give one investigation to confirm your answer to question 1:
    a) Renal ultrasound
    b) Renal angiogram
    c) Urine dipstick plus microscopy
    d) Urine microscopy and eosinophil count
    e) PTH level
    f) Renal biopsy
    g) Vitamin D level

3. Give one specific management for your answer to question 1:
    a) Alkalinization of urine
    b) Stop NSAIDs
    c) Fluid restrict
    d) ACE inhibition
    e) Intravenous calcium gluconate

Case 1.9

A 35-year-old alcoholic was found lying in the gutter unconscious. He looked malnourished, with nicotine-stained fingers, bilateral Dupuytren's contractures and several spider naevi. His temperature was 36.8 °C, respiratory rate 24/min, blood pressure 100/60 mmHg, and pulse 80/min. Heart sounds were normal, as were chest and abdominal examinations. There was no facial or skull bruising and no neck stiffness. His GCS was 5. He extended his limbs to pain. Pupils were equal at 4 mm. Pupillary and corneal reflexes were normal. His eyes were dysconjugate, but oculocephalic reflexes were intact. Limb tone was increased, with brisk reflexes and bilateral up-going plantars. Finger-prick glucose was 3.6 mmol/l. No response to

50 ml 50% dextrose. Urea and electrolytes were normal. He remained unconscious throughout the next 24 hours. CT head scan was normal.

1. What is the most likely diagnosis?
    a) Brainstem infarct
    b) Hepatic encephalopathy
    c) Herpes simplex encephalitis
    d) Post-alcoholic seizure
    e) Subarachnoid haemorrhage
    f) Overdose

Case 1.10

A 50-year-old lady presented with a one-month history of fatigue and depression. She had lost her appetite and had noticed some weight loss. She complained that the shape of objects appeared distorted and out of alignment. On examination she appeared depressed, but examination was otherwise normal. Full blood count, electrolytes, calcium, phosphate, thyroid function and immunoglobulins were all normal. Syphilis and HIV serology were negative. She was commenced on fluoxetine. On review one month later, she was brought into the clinic with the assistance of her husband. She claimed to be unable to see and needed guiding to her chair. Her husband reported that she was extremely apathetic and generally unable to perform any of her normal daily tasks. On examination she sat silently, displaying little spontaneous activity except for occasional jerking of her limbs. However, she did exhibit a marked startle response to an unexpected hand-clap. Attempts at higher mental function testing were limited to three- and four-word responses, most of which were inappropriate. She said she could not see any of the picture boards. However, fundoscopy and pupillary reactions were normal. The remainder of the cranial nerve examination was normal. Limb power seemed intact, with normal reflexes but bilateral up-going plantars. General examination was normal.

CT was normal. CSF: no cells, protein 0.4 g/l, no oligoclonal bands.

1. What is the most likely diagnosis?
    a) Variant Creutzfeldt–Jakob disease (vCJD)
    b) Creutzfeldt–Jakob disease (CJD)
    c) Fluoxetine side effect
    d) Huntington's chorea
    e) Lithium intoxication
    f) Alzheimer's disease with myoclonus
    g) Depressive stupor
    h) Limbic encephalitis

Exam 2

████

Case 2.1

A 77-year-old retired cabinetmaker was seen in the urgent assessment clinic with a slow-to-resolve pneumonia. His GP had requested a CXR after symptoms had persisted despite a course of oral antibiotics. This was reported as showing 'collapse/consolidation of the right upper zone with a suggestion of increased density at the right hilum'. The patient himself was vague about his history, saying he had suffered with wheezy bronchitis since his teens, and more recently with a regular winter pneumonia. He smoked 20 cigarettes per day. When asked about his medication, he emptied a plastic bag full of an assortment of inhalers and a nasal spray on to the clinic desk, admitting to using them only when he felt it necessary. A repeat CXR now showed additionally some left perihilar consolidation.

Na 132 mmol/l, K 4.6 mmol/l, urea 9.7 mmol/l, creatinine 132 μmol/l, Hb 14.8 g/dl, white cell count 14.2×10^9/l (neutrophils 8.3×10^9/l, lymphocytes 2.4×10^9/l), platelets 356×10^9/l.

1. What is the most likely diagnosis?
   a) Allergic bronchopulmonary aspergillosis (ABPA)
   b) Hypersensitivity pneumonitis (woodworker's lung)
   c) Churg–Strauss syndrome
   d) *Mycoplasma* pneumonia
   e) Bronchoalveolar carcinoma

2. Choose the best of the following options for further investigation:
   a) High-resolution chest CT and bronchoalveolar lavage with transbronchial biopsy
   b) ANCA determination and bronchoalveolar lavage with transbronchial biopsy
   c) High-resolution chest CT and precipitins against wood dust and *Alternaria* antigens
   d) High-resolution chest CT and *Aspergillus* skin prick test
   e) Mycoplasma IgM ELISA and cold agglutinin determination

Case 2.2

A 48-year-old man with poorly controlled diabetes presented with a five-day history of increasingly severe right-sided facial pain, fever and blocked nose. On examination he was very dehydrated, confused and slightly drowsy. His temperature was 39.2 °C. There was swelling over the right maxilla with slight erythema, and unilateral nasal obstruction with a necrotic inferior turbinate. Palatal ulceration was evident. There was no proptosis.

Hb 13.6 g/dl, white cell count 20.4 × 10^9/l. Blood glucose 44 mmol/l. Urine ketones +++. Standard diabetic ketoacidosis management was initiated.

1. What is the most likely diagnosis?
   a) Poorly controlled diabetes, bacterial sinusitis, and cavernous sinus thrombosis
   b) Diabetes and Wegener's granulomatosis
   c) Diabetes and necrotizing fasciitis
   d) Poorly controlled diabetes and rhinocerebral mucorycosis
   e) Poorly controlled diabetes, bacterial sinusitis, and subdural empyema

2. Select the next step:
   a) Multiple blood cultures, head CT, and empirical broad-spectrum antibacterial agents
   b) Head CT, CSF analysis, and empirical broad-spectrum antibacterial agents
   c) Head CT, surgical debridement and urgent histology, and intravenous amphotericin B
   d) Head CT, cANCA, CXR, urinalysis, and intravenous steroids
   e) Head CT, surgical debridement, and broad-spectrum antibacterial agents

Case 2.3

A 60-year-old man had his congenitally bicuspid valve replaced uneventfully with a mechanical prosthesis. Six weeks post-surgery, he developed recurrent fevers. On examination he was febrile at 38.4 °C, with a clinical small left-sided pleural effusion and soft systolic murmur in the aortic area. No other abnormality was found. In particular, there was no regurgitant murmur, the prosthetic closing sound was crisp, and there were no stigmata of infective endocarditis.

CXR: small left pleural effusion, valve prosthesis. Transthoracic echo: well-sited prosthetic valve. Moderate pericardial effusion, but no evidence of tamponade. Repeat blood cultures: no growth. MSU: no growth. Sputum culture: no growth. ECG: first-degree heart block, low voltages generally.

1. Select the three statements from the following that are most appropriate to the clinical scenario:
   a) Transfusion-associated CMV infection is the likely diagnosis
   b) Potential complications include constrictive pericarditis and pericardial tamponade
   c) Peroperative infection with an organism of low virulence, such as a coagulase-negative *Staphylococcus*, is most likely
   d) Immediate pericardial aspiration for culture is mandatory

e) 10–20% of patients may experience a similar syndrome after cardiac surgery
f) Intravenous vancomycin would be appropriate empirical therapy
g) Treatment with NSAIDs is likely to lead to rapid clinical resolution
h) First-degree heart block is strong evidence for an aortic root abscess
i) Ultimately, a repeat aortic valve replacement is likely to be necessary

Case 2.4

A 30-year-old Indian restaurant employee presented with a four-month history of fevers. He felt quite well and had sought medical attention only on account of weight loss. He had no relevant past medical or family history. On examination he was thin and pale, with palpable lymph nodes in his axillae, cervical chain and groin. He had 4-cm smooth hepatomegaly and 15-cm splenomegaly. There were no stigmata of chronic liver disease. His ankles were swollen, but cardiovascular and respiratory examinations were otherwise normal. His temperature was 38.2 °C.

Hb 6.6 g/dl, white cell count 1.8×10^9/l, platelets 100×10^9/l. Film: normochromic, normocytic anaemia. No malaria parasites on three separate thick and thin films. Albumin 22 g/l, total protein 70 g/l.

1. Select the most likely diagnosis from the following:
   a) Chronic brucellosis
   b) Non-Hodgkin's lymphoma
   c) Tropical splenomegaly syndrome
   d) Visceral leishmaniasis
   e) *Schistosoma mansoni* infection
   f) Miliary tuberculosis

2. Which of the following investigations is likely to be diagnostic?
   a) Leishmanin skin test
   b) Heaf test
   c) Histological examination of bone marrow aspirate
   d) Histological examination of rectal biopsy
   e) Prolonged culture of blood

Case 2.5

A man presents with a novel neurological syndrome. The extended family are traced and examined:

1. What is the likely mode of inheritance?
   a) Autosomal dominant

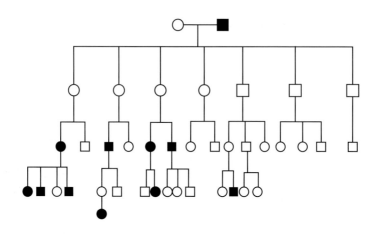

b) Autosomal recessive
c) Maternal genomic imprinting
d) Mitochondrial transmission
e) Paternal genomic imprinting
f) X-linked dominant
g) X-linked recessive
h) Y-linked

Case 2.6

A 44-year-old lady presented six months previously with a three-week history of abdominal pain, malaise, fevers and diarrhoea. Diagnosis was hastened by her development of small bowel obstruction. At operation, a stricture together with 30 cm of inflamed terminal ileum were removed. Since the operation she had generally felt well but had been troubled by persistent diarrhoea. This was non-bloody, not foul-smelling, and tended to be worse in the morning. She had no abdominal pain.

Full blood count and electrolytes: normal. ESR 15 mm/h, CRP 6 mg/l. White cell scan: normal. Serum B_{12} 200 ng/l, red cell folate 300 µg/l. Abdominal X-ray: normal.

1. Which further test is most likely to lead to the correct diagnosis?
   a) ^{75}Se-homotaurocholic acid test
   b) Fasting gut hormones
   c) ^{14}C-xylose breath test
   d) Upper gastrointestinal endoscopy and duodenal biopsy
   e) ^{111}In-labelled white cell scan

2. What treatment would you give?
   a) Cholestyramine
   b) High-dose oral proton pump inhibitors
   c) Prolonged course of co-trimoxazole (at least one year)

    d) Oral metronidazole and amoxicillin
    e) Oral 5-aminosalicylate derivative

Case 2.7

A 40-year-old smelter was found by the nurse at the preoperative assessment clinic to have protein and glucose on urine dipstick. He was therefore referred for a medical opinion. Apart from an inguinal hernia, a right Colles' fracture and some breathlessness, he was well with no past medical or family history. He took occasional paracetamol for headaches but no other medication and had never smoked. Examination revealed hyperexpanded lungs with occasional diffuse inspiratory crepitations. No other abnormality was detected. His blood pressure was 110/70 mmHg.

Na 136 mmol/l, K 3.3 mmol/l, urea 5.9 mmol/l, creatinine 130 µmol/l, albumin 38 g/l, urate 0.15 mmol/l, glucose 4.2 mmol/l. Immunoglobulins, electrophoresis, C3 and C4: all normal. ANAs, anti-dsDNA antibodies: negative. Urine dipstick: protein and glucose. Urine microscopy: normal. CXR: emphysematous changes. IVP: normal. Urine osmolality after overnight fast: 900 mmol/kg.

1. Select the most likely underlying problem:
    a) Heavy-metal poisoning
    b) Multiple myeloma
    c) Analgesic nephropathy
    d) AL amyloidosis
    e) Wilson's disease

Case 2.8

A 65-year-old man presented with a two-month history of increasing lethargy and weakness. At times he felt dizzy, and once he briefly lost vision in one eye. He was admitted to hospital following a nosebleed but then developed a DVT whilst an in-patient.

His fundal appearance is shown below:

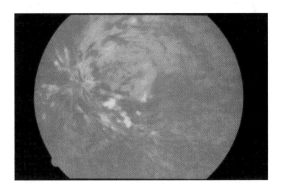

1. Which description of this appearance fits best?
   a) Diabetic retinopathy
   b) Hypertensive retinopathy
   c) Papilloedema
   d) Central retinal artery occlusion
   e) Central retinal vein occlusion

Neurological examination was otherwise normal. Pulse was 90/min and regular. Blood pressure was 140/80 mmHg with no drop. A 1-cm liver edge and spleen tip were palpable. The remainder of the examination was normal.

Hb 9.7 g/dl, white cell count 10.3 × 10^9/l, platelets 170 × 10^9/l, PT 12 s (normal: 10–12 s), APTT 30 s (normal: 30–35 s), ESR 80 mm/h, urea 13.7 mmol/l, creatinine 130 μmol/l, calcium 2.6 mmol/l, phosphate 1.3 mmol/l. Arterial blood gases: pO$_2$ 13.3 kPa, pCO$_2$ 4.3 kPa, pH 7.34.

2. Suggest the most likely underlying diagnosis:
   a) Non-Hodgkin's lymphoma with brain metastases
   b) Hodgkin's lymphoma with brain metastases
   c) Sarcoidosis
   d) Myeloma
   e) Waldenström's macroglobulinaemia
   f) Haemochromatosis

3. Select the best investigation from the following to confirm your diagnosis:
   a) CT head scan
   b) Blood film
   c) Splenic aspirate
   d) Gallium scan
   e) Kveim test
   f) Broncheoalveolar lavage
   g) Serum and CSF ACE levels
   h Plasma immunoglobulins and electrophoresis
   i) Liver biopsy

Case 2.9

A 70-year-old lady was found stuck in her armchair at her nursing home. She said that over the previous few weeks she had found it increasingly difficult to rise from her chair and walking was a struggle. On examination she had marked proximal muscle weakness, affecting mainly the lower limbs. Reflexes, co-ordination and sensation were normal, although the ankle jerks were absent. Both plantars were down-going. The remainder of the neurological examination was normal. Apart from an ejection systolic murmur, the general examination was entirely normal.

Hb 10.7 g/dl, white cell count 4.5×10^9/l, platelets 330×10^9/l, MCV 104 fl, Na 136 mmol/l, K 4.4 mmol/l, urea 5.6 mmol/l, creatinine 105 μmol/l, glucose 8.5 mmol/l.

1. Select three possible causes for the weakness:
   a) Alcoholic myopathy
   b) Diabetic amyotrophy
   c) Hypothyroidism
   d) Polymyositis
   e) Limb girdle dystrophy
   f) Osteomalacia
   g) Dystrophia myotonica
   h) Diabetes mellitus
   i) Myasthenia gravis

2. Select four investigations from the following that you would carry out:
   a) TSH/T$_4$
   b) Alcohol history
   c) EMG
   d) Serum calcium
   e) B$_{12}$, folate
   f) Muscle biopsy
   g) Vitamin D levels
   h) Tensilon test
   i) Acetylcholine receptor antibody

Case 2.10

A 44-year-old man presented with a long history of troublesome episodic sweating, flushing and weakness, which seemed to occur after meals. His past medical history included asthma, hay fever, and a vagotomy and pyloroplasty ten years previously for a gastric ulcer resistant to the then available medications. His mother had thyroid problems. Examination was entirely normal.

1. Which investigation would you arrange next?
   a) 24-hour urinary 5-hydroxyindoleacetate levels
   b) Genetic analysis of the *menin* gene
   c) Radiolabelled octreotide scintigraphy
   d) Five-hour oral glucose tolerance test with insulin levels
   e) Abdominal CT imaging with contrast

Exam 3

Case 3.1

A 58-year-old lorry driver had been suffering from intermittent left-sided chest pain for several months. More recently this was associated with left shoulder and arm ache. He noticed he was becoming more breathless when unloading his lorry. He smoked 30 cigarettes per day and had a long-standing smoker's cough. On examination expansion was decreased at the left base with dullness to percussion and decreased breath sounds. The chest radiograph is shown below:

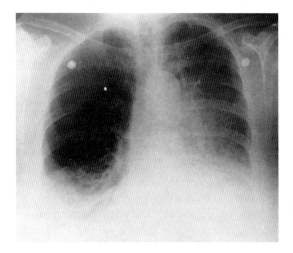

1. What does the chest radiograph show?
    a) No abnormalities
    b) Signs of left lower lobe collapse
    c) Signs of left lower lobe alveolar disease
    d) Signs of left upper lobe collapse
    e) Signs of left upper lobe alveolar disease

ECG and bronchoscopy were normal. Fluoroscopy revealed paradoxical left hemidiaphragmatic movement. One week later he presented as an emergency with increasing shortness of breath. He was afebrile, but the brachial pulse was faint and at a rate of 120/min. Blood pressure was 90/60 mmHg. The JVP was raised. Chest signs were unchanged. Heart sounds were normal but quiet.

2. What is the most likely diagnosis?
   a) Lingular pneumonia with septic shock
   b) Cardiac tamponade due to bronchial carcinoma in the lingular segment of the left upper lobe
   c) Acute-on-chronic pulmonary embolism
   d) Left-sided tension pneumothorax secondary to bronchial carcinoma
   e) Cardiac tamponade due to bronchial carcinoma in the left lower lobe

Case 3.2

A 24-year-old postdoctoral fellow returned from a conference in the USA one week previously with increasing breathlessness and fever. He had missed the last three days of lectures to go camping in Arizona. He was working on transgenic mice. On examination he looked ill. His temperature was 38.7 °C, pulse was 120/min and blood pressure was 100/50 mmHg. His JVP was not seen and his heart sounds were normal. There was no peripheral oedema, rash or arthropathy. His respiratory rate was 30/min, with a saturation of 84% on a rebreathing mask. Crepitations were audible throughout both lung fields.

CXR showed bilateral alveolar shadowing. Heart size normal. ECG normal. After admission to ICU, intubation and catheter placement, an adult respiratory distress syndrome (ARDS)-like picture was confirmed. Microscopy and immunofluorescence of lavaged material revealed no signs of infection, including specifically *Coxiella burnetti*, influenza, parainfluenza, *Chlamydia psittaci*, *Mycoplasma pneumoniae*, *Pneumocystis* and *Histoplasma*. Urine *Legionella* antigen was negative.

1. Select the most likely diagnosis from the following:
   a) Coccidioidomycosis
   b) Hantavirus infection
   c) Histoplasmosis
   d) Bronchiolitis obliterans with organizing pneumonia
   e) Respiratory syncytial virus infection

2. What specific treatment would you start?
   a) Amphotericin B
   b) Itraconazole
   c) Ribavirin
   d) High-dose corticosteroids
   e) None

Case 3.3

On the day before a 19-year-old student was due to fly to Nairobi for summer vacation, he developed abdominal and lumbar pain. He managed to see his GP the following morning, by which time he was jaundiced with dark urine. He was pale and icteric, but otherwise examination was normal.

Hb 7.8 g/dl, white cell count 11×10^9/l, platelets 250×10^9/l.

1. What is the diagnosis?
   a) Paroxysmal nocturnal haemoglobinuria
   b) Sickle cell anaemia with acute sequestration syndrome
   c) G6PD deficiency
   d) Adenoma of the ampulla of Vater
   e) Beta-thalassaemia trait and biliary colic

2. Choose the investigation from the following that is most likely to be helpful:
   a) Ham's test
   b) Serum G6PD assay
   c) Abdominal ultrasound examination
   d) HbA2 determination
   e) Blood film
   f) Clotting studies

Case 3.4

A 24-year-old medical student presented with a seven-day history of fevers, sweats and right shoulder tip pain. There were no other complaints. He had spent much of his elective in South Africa two months previously, travelling in rural areas. Percussion over the lower costal cartilages was painful, and breath sounds were reduced at the right base. Examination was otherwise normal. ALP 150 U/l, liver function tests otherwise normal. CXR: raised right hemidiaphragm.

1. What is the most likely diagnosis?
   a) Ascending cholangitis due to *Salmonella typhi*
   b) Right subphrenic abscess
   c) Amoebic dysentery
   d) Right lower lobe pneumonia
   e) Tuberculosis
   f) Hepatic amoebic abscess
   g) Hepatic *Streptococcus milleri* abscess

2. Choose the next two investigations from the following:
   a) Liver ultrasound

b) *Entamoeba histolytica* serology
c) Microscopy of wet-mounted fresh stool sample
d) Rectal biopsy
e) Repeated blood cultures
f) Heaf test
g) Bronchoscopy and lavage
h) Guided aspiration of any hepatic abscess

Case 3.5

A 35-year-old man was referred with abnormal facial movements and uncontrollable limb twitches, which had been building up over several months. He had been
an in-patient at the local psychiatric hospital for the previous two years, and he had
recently been started on a new medication. His notes said that a cousin had also
ended up in psychiatric care. His parents died in a car crash when he was a child. On
examination his mouth and lips were intermittently contorted and his arms would
move from one abnormal posture to another. Cranial nerve examination was normal
and he had no long tract signs. Peripheral nervous system was intact. General examination was normal.

Hb 9.4 g/dl, white cell count 4.5×10^9/l, platelets 330×10^9/l, Na 138 mmol/l,
K 4.4 mmol/l, urea 3.5 mmol/l, creatinine 80 μmol/l, bicarbonate 15 mmol/l, chloride
110 mmol/l, glucose 4.5 mmol/l.

1. What is the most likely diagnosis?
   a) Huntington's chorea
   b) Wilson's disease
   c) Neuroleptic-induced dyskinesia
   d) Thyrotoxicosis
   e) Sydenham's chorea
   f) Antiphospholipid syndrome

Case 3.6

A 27-year-old management consultant presented to the surgeons with sudden-onset
abdominal pain that was worse on movement. Her bowels had been opening regularly with a normal stool. She was nauseated but did not vomit. She had been completely well until one hour previously, with an unremarkable past medical and family
history. She was on the pill and took occasional herbal tonics to help her through
her stressful day. On examination she was pale with cold peripheries. There were
no stigmata of chronic liver disease. Her pulse was 130/min, blood pressure
was 80/40 mmHg, and heart sounds were normal. She had a tender abdomen, with

guarding and rebound tenderness in the right upper quadrant. The right hepatic lobe was palpable.

Hb 7.5 g/dl. Electrolytes, liver function, amylase, CXR and abdominal X-ray: all normal.

1. Choose the diagnosis from the following that fits best:
   a) Acute intermittent porphyric attack precipitated by oestrogen
   b) Thrombosis of hepatic vein
   c) Hepatic infarction
   d) Lead poisoning
   e) Acute cholecystitis
   f) Aortic dissection
   g) Haemorrhage into hepatic adenoma

2. Which of the following would *not* be diagnostically helpful?
   a) MRI
   b) Ultrasonography
   c) ^{99m}Tc-scintigraphy
   d) Blood cultures
   e) Angiography

3. Which of the following would be the most appropriate step towards definitive management?
   a) Percutaneous biopsy
   b) Laparotomy
   c) Intravenous heparin
   d) Blood lead determination
   e) Urinary porphobilinogen determination

Case 3.7

An 18-year-old student presented with a two-month history of fatigue, weakness, nausea and vomiting. Since the age of five he had wet the bed, and he always seemed to drink and urinate more than his taller sister. On examination he was pale and of short stature. He had a waddling gait, with signs of a proximal myopathy. His pulse was 100/min. Blood pressure was 100/60 mmHg when lying down and 70/40 mmHg when standing. His JVP was not seen. Heart sounds were normal. Knock-knees were evident.

Hb 7.4 g/dl, white cell count 5.5×10^9/l, platelets 160×10^9/l, Na 137 mmol/l, K 4.8 mmol/l, urea 55 mmol/l, creatinine 598 μmol/l, calcium 1.6 mmol/l, phosphate 2.5 mmol/l, ALP 240 U/l. IVP showed small, irregular kidneys with normal pelvicalyceal systems and bladder. Skeletal survey showed bone age of 14, subperiosteal phalangeal erosions, increased density of vertebral endplates, and widened epiphyses of long bones with poorly defined metaphyses. With sodium supplements, his creatinine clearance rose from 2 ml/min to 10 ml/min and his postural drop disappeared.

1. What is the most likely diagnosis?
    a) Medullary cystic disease
    b) Medullary sponge kidney
    c) Autosomal recessive polycystic kidney disease
    d) Type 1 vitamin D dependent rickets
    e) Reflux nephropathy

Case 3.8

A 26-year-old joiner presented with a 36-hour history of increasingly severe abdominal pain associated with back pain and rigors. He felt nauseated and had vomited once. His bowels were opening normally. He had been feeling more tired than usual for several weeks preceding his admission. On examination he was febrile at 38.9 °C and looked very ill and dehydrated. Pulse was 120/min. Blood pressure was 100/60 mmHg when lying down and 80/40 mmHg when sitting. He was tender in his epigastrium and right upper quadrant, with guarding in the right upper quadrant. There was a suggestion of a mass under the area of guarding. Bowel sounds and rectal examination were both normal. The remainder of the examination was normal.

Hb 12.8 g/dl, white cell count 27.4 × 10⁹/l (90% neutrophils), platelets 440 × 10⁹/l, Na 134 mmol/l, K 5.4 mmol/l, urea 25 mmol/l, creatinine 170 μmol/l, serum osmolality 350 mosmol/kg, ALT 30 U/l, bilirubin 25 μmol/l, ALP 180 U/l, INR 1.2. Urine microscopy, ECG and CXR were all normal.

A detail of the plain abdominal X-ray is shown below:

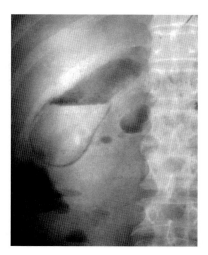

1. Which one or more of the following radiographic features is/are shown?
   a) Normal appearance
   b) Mucosal oedema at the hepatic flexure
   c) Gallstones
   d) Rigler's sign
   e) Gas in the gallbladder wall
   f) Gas in the bowel wall
   g) Porcelain gallbladder

2. Select the two diagnoses from the following that best fit this scenario:
   a) Type 2 lactic acidosis
   b) Polyarteritis nodosum
   c) Bowel infarction
   d) Emphysematous cholecystitis
   e) Diabetic ketoacidosis
   f) Ethylene glycol poisoning
   g) Hepatic abscess
   h) Ascending cholangitis
   i) Pancreatitis

Case 3.9

A 60-year-old lady from Syria presented with rigors and presyncope. No further history was available. On examination she was febrile at 38.5 °C and flushed. Her pulse was 120/min. Blood pressure was 120/80 mmHg when lying down and 100/60 mmHg when sitting. Her JVP was not visible and heart sounds were normal. Her chest was clear. A left paramedian abdominal scar was evident, together with a tender right flank. There was no neurological abnormality as far as it was possible to assess.

Hb 13.4 g/dl, white cell count 18.9×10^9/l, platelets 447×10^9/l, PT 13 s (normal: 10–12 s), Na 144 mmol/l, K 2.9 mm/l, urea 10.4 mmol/l, creatinine 140 μmol/l, chloride 118 mmol/l, bicarbonate 13 mmol/l. No urine was available for analysis.

1. Select the two most likely diagnoses from the following:
   a) Diabetic ketoacidosis (DKA)
   b) Acute renal failure
   c) Right-sided pyelonephritis
   d) Malignant bowel perforation with tracking of bowel contents down right paracolic gutter
   e) Ureterosigmoidostomy
   f) Type 2 renal tubular acidosis
   g) Pancreatitis
   h) Haemorrhage into metastatic neuroendocrine tumour

Case 3.10

A 55-year-old lady presented with flushing attacks. Initially these lasted only minutes, but each attack now lasted hours. She often felt wheezy at the height of each flush and would lacrimate. On direct questioning her stools had been loose recently and her menses had been irregular for the previous two years. Her sister had a peanut allergy. Her facial appearance is shown below:

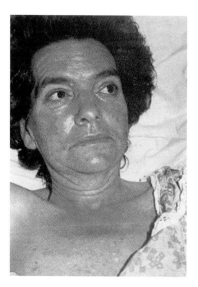

Blood pressure was 110/80 mmHg with no postural drop. Her apex beat was undisplaced and of normal character. Her JVP was not raised. An ejection systolic murmur was audible in the aortic area, radiating into the carotids and loudest on expiration. There was no ankle oedema. Respiratory and abdominal examinations were normal.

Hb 10.4 g/dl, white cell count 4×10^9/l, platelets 380×10^9/l. Electrolytes and liver function tests were normal. Ultrasound of abdomen: normal liver and spleen, no masses seen.

1. Choose the single most accurate diagnosis from the following:
    a) Appendiceal carcinoid tumour
    b) Bronchial carcinoid tumour
    c) Systemic mastocytosis
    d) Phaeochromocytoma
    e) Verner–Morrison syndrome
    f) Climacteric flushes

2. Select the most helpful investigation from each of the three groups below:

   a) Small-bowel enteroscopy
   b) Octreotide scintigraphy
   c) Serum tryptase

   d) Urinary histamine metabolites
   e) MIBG scan
   f) Abdominal CT

   g) Fasting gut hormones
   h) Spiral CT chest
   i) Plasma catecholamines

Exam 4

Case 4.1

A 23-year-old unemployed mother of three presented with a ten-day history of progressive breathlessness, dry cough, fever and malaise. By the time of her admission she was barely able to move. She admitted to no previous history. Her husband was a foundry worker and pigeon fancier in his spare time. On examination she was cyanosed but not clubbed. Her temperature was 37.7 °C, pulse was 130/min, and blood pressure was 120/70 mmHg. Heart sounds were normal, JVP was normal, and there was no peripheral oedema. Widespread inspiratory crepitations were audible.

Hb 13. 4 g/dl, white cell count 14.2 × 10⁹/l (neutrophils 85%, lymphocytes 14%), platelets 230 × 10⁹/l, PT 12 s (normal: 12–14 s), ESR 80 mm/h, pO_2 5.0 kPa, pCO_2 2.8 kPa, pH 7.37. No growth from induced sputum. Mantoux (1/100 tuberculin) negative. Blood cultures negative. Influenza A and B, parainfluenza, adenovirus, *Coxiella burnetti*, *Mycoplasma* and *Chlamydia psittaci*: initial titres negative. KCO 60% predicted. The plain chest radiograph was reported to show bilateral, diffuse and poorly defined alveolar shadowing.

1. From the list below, select the two most likely diagnoses:
   a) Pneumocystis carinii pneumonia in HIV
   b) Sarcoidosis
   c) Hamman–Rich syndrome
   d) Atypical pneumonia
   e) Miliary tuberculosis
   f) Pigeon fancier's lung
   g) Pulmonary haemorrhage
   h) Allergic bronchopulmonary aspergillosis
   i) Acute idiopathic eosinophilic pneumonia

2. Which two of the following investigations would be *unlikely* to help?
   a) Serum avian precipitins
   b) HIV test with consent
   c) Serum ACE
   d) Bronchoscopy and lavage/biopsy
   e) ANCA determination

Case 4.2

A 43-year-old long-term homeless man is admitted with vague symptoms of headache, leg cramps, malaise and loss of weight over several weeks. Although difficult to define his intake exactly, it is clear that he does abuse alcohol, but there is no evidence of intravenous drug use or other risk factors for bloodborne viral infection. The only past medical history obtained is of treatment for cellulitis two years previously.

Barrier precautions are observed for examination due to a heavy infestation by lice of both head and body. He appears malnourished and unkempt, with numerous excoriations on his trunk and limbs. His temperature is 38.1 °C. There is a marked purpuric rash over the extremities, as well as several conjunctival haemorrhages. The circulation is hyperdynamic and there is moderate hepatojugular reflux. A long early diastolic murmur is audible in expiration at the left sternal edge, and there are fine crepitations at both lung bases as well as mild ankle oedema bilaterally.

Hb 11.9 g/dl, platelets 95 × 10⁹/l, white cell count 11 × 10⁹/l (neutrophils 70%, lymphocytes 29%), clotting normal, ESR 78 mm/h, CRP 48 mg/l, Na 134 mmol/l, K 4.5 mmol/l, urea 8.1 mmol/l, creatinine 150 µmol/l, albumin 29 g/l, ALT 50 IU/l, GGT 170 U/l, ALP 205 IU/l, bilirubin 16 µmol/l. HBV, HCV and HIV serology: all negative. Rheumatoid factor weakly positive. ANA, ANCA and cryoglobulins: all negative. Urinalysis: protein ++, blood +++. Transthoracic echocardiogram: moderate to severe aortic regurgitation with the suggestion of a mass on the non-coronary cusp. Blood cultures negative on 12 occasions from different sites, each after two days' growth.

1. Select the most likely diagnosis:
   a) *Bartonella quintana* endocarditis
   b) Atrial myxoma
   c) Non-infective endocarditis
   d) Fungal endocarditis
   e) Whipple's disease
   f) Chronic brucellosis
   g) *Mycoplasma pneumoniae* endocarditis

2. Choose the best empirical treatment from the following:
   a) Immediate surgery and histology of excised aortic valve
   b) Intravenous vancomycin
   c) Intravenous vancomycin and gentamicin
   d) Intravenous penicillin and gentamicin
   e) Intravenous erythromycin and gentamicin
   f) Corticosteroids

Case 4.3

An 18-year-old student who was not sporty at school decided to take up rowing at university. He found that he would develop fatigue and weakness about ten minutes into his rowing, symptoms that would last several minutes before wearing off, despite continued rowing. At first he thought this was just lack of fitness, but his symptoms persisted despite adhering to his fitness programme. After his first race he passed very dark urine, precipitating his appointment with the doctor. Examination was normal.

1. Select the most likely diagnosis from the list below:
   a) Lipid metabolism defect
   b) McArdle's disease
   c) Metabolic myopathy
   d) Hypokalaemic periodic paralysis
   e) Hyperkalaemic periodic paralysis

2. Select the most pertinent investigation from the following:
   a) EMG
   b) Triglyceride subtype levels
   c) Muscle biopsy
   d) Ischaemic forearm exercise test
   e) Serum potassium

Case 4.4

A 24-year-old unemployed woman presented to the surgeons with a 24-hour history of diffuse severe abdominal pain radiating around to her back. She was anorexic and nauseated and had vomited twice. Her bowels had not opened for three days, although she was passing flatus. She had recently been depressed, but she had no other past medical history. She was sweaty, with a blood pressure of 160/100 mmHg and pulse of 130/min. Her abdomen was diffusely tender, but there was no guarding and bowel sounds were normal. Examination was otherwise normal. She was made nil by mouth, given an intravenous drip and given intramuscular morphine for her pain. Full blood count, electrolytes, CXR and abdominal X-ray were all normal. One hour after her injection, she complained of being unable to raise her arms on account of weakness and breathlessness. A neurologist was called promptly.

1. Select the best diagnosis from the following:
   a) Salmonella poisoning
   b) Acute intermittent porphyria (AIP)
   c) Paroxysmal nocturnal haemoglobinuria (PNH)
   d) Acute brachial neuritis
   e) Guillain-Barré syndrome
   f) Phaeochromocytoma

elect three investigations from the following that you would carry out:
a) Peak flow
b) Vital capacity
c) Urinary porphobilinogen and aminolaevulinic acid
d) Blood film
e) Ham's test
f) Plasma catecholamines
g) Nerve conduction studies

Case 4.5

A 45-year-old man was referred to a urologist with nocturnal incontinence. Six times in the previous six months he had awoken in a wet bed, not having consumed excess fluid or alcohol the previous night. Bladder function during the day was normal. He had no past medical history. Examination was normal. Full blood count and electrolytes were normal.

1. Which of the following is the most likely diagnosis?
   a) Urinary sphincter dyssynergia
   b) Interstitial cystitis
   c) Epilepsy
   d) Alzheimer's disease
   e) Diabetes mellitus
   f) Diabetes insipidus

2. Select two investigations from the following:
   a) EEG
   b) CT head
   c) IVP
   d) CXR
   e) Micturating cystogram
   f) Cystoscopy
   g) Nocturnal blood glucose
   h) Nocturnal urinary glucose
   i) Serum osmolality
   j) Urine osmolality

Case 4.6

A 26-year-old secretary presented with abdominal pain, nausea and vomiting following a four-day flu-like prodrome. He had no past medical history, took no medications and had undertaken no recent foreign travel. On examination he was jaundiced, with a palpable liver edge.

ALT 1200 U/l, ALP 330 U/l, bilirubin 120 μmol/l. Anti-hepatitis A IgM was raised. Anti-hepatitis B core IgM antibody and hepatitis B surface antigen were not detected. On follow-up in clinic two months later, he felt better. However, his ALT was 75 U/l, ALP was 160 U/l and bilirubin was 70 μmol/l, and therefore another four-month appointment was made. His ALT was then 36 U/l, albumin 40 g/l, ALP 110 U/l and bilirubin 40 μmol/l. Haptoglobins were normal. Apart from slight jaundice, examination was normal.

1. What is the most likely diagnosis?
    a) Hepatitis C infection
    b) Chronic active hepatitis
    c) Gilbert's syndrome
    d) *Cryptosporidium* infection
    e) Chronic extravascular haemolysis

2. Which of the following investigations is appropriate next?
    a) Unconjugated bilirubin levels
    b) Serum electrophoresis
    c) Liver biopsy
    d) Liver ultrasound
    e) Anti-hepatitis C IgG
    f) Anti-smooth muscle and liver/kidney microsomal antibodies

Case 4.7

A 20-year-old medical student discovered a lump in his neck during the pathology course. His friends dismissed him as neurotic, but he decided to seek proper advice two weeks later when his ankles began to swell. Apart from perennial rhinitis and asthma, he had no previous medical problems. On examination an enlarged lymph node was palpable in the right cervical chain. There were no signs of local infection. His pulse was 80/min and blood pressure was 120/80 mmHg. The JVP was not raised and heart sounds were normal. There was no organomegaly. His face and ankles were swollen.

Full blood count and electrolytes were normal. Albumin 24 g/l, ALT 22 U/l. Urine dipstick: protein +++. Microscopy of urine was normal. Light microscopy of renal biopsy was normal.

1. Choose the single most likely diagnosis from each of the two groups below:
    a) Tuberculosis
    b) Cat scratch disease
    c) Hodgkin's disease

d) Sarcoidosis
e) Diabetes

f) Focal segmental glomerulosclerosis (FSGS)
g) Minimal change glomerulonephropathy (MCN)
h) Membranous glomerulonephritis
i) Proximal renal tubular dysfunction
j) Glomerular hyperfiltration

2. Choose the next two steps to take:
   a) Electron microscopy of renal biopsy
   b) Serum ACE
   c) Lymph node biopsy
   d) CXR
   e) CT abdomen and pelvis
   f) Renal ultrasound
   g) Serum cholesterol
   h) Serial early-morning urine specimens for mycobacterial microscopy and culture
   i) *Bartonella* serology
   j) Oral glucose tolerance test

Case 4.8

A 30-year-old man presented with a five-year history of increasing weakness and stiffness of his lower limbs. More recently, he had noticed some frequency and urgency of micturition and was having problem maintaining an erection. He occasionally felt faint but had no other symptoms. His past medical history was unremarkable and there was no family history. He was taking no medications, smoked ten cigarettes per day and drank alcohol only occasionally. Higher mental function, cranial nerve and upper limb examinations were normal. Tone was increased bilaterally in the lower limbs with grade 4/5 pyramidal weakness, brisk reflexes and up-going plantars. Vibration sense was absent to the knees. There was no ataxia. His blood pressure was 120/80 mmHg when down lying and 100/60 mmHg when standing. He appeared pigmented, but examination was otherwise normal.

Hb 13.5 g/dl, white cell count 4.5×10^9/l, platelets 340×10^9/l, Na 128 mmol/l, K 5.4 mmol/l, urea 4.5 mmol/l, creatinine 77 μmol/l.

1. What is the most likely diagnosis?
   a) Whipple's disease
   b) Coeliac disease
   c) Sarcoidosis
   d) Adrenoleukodystrophy

e) Vitamin E deficiency
f) Vitamin B12 deficiency

Case 4.9

A 75-year-old man was reviewed in clinic following a recent chest infection. This was his third chest infection within six months, and he complained that even when not feverish he seemed to be coughing up a lot of green sputum. He also thought he was getting more breathless generally and sometimes felt faint when standing up. He had no chest pain or palpitation and had noticed no blood. Prior to this year he had been fit and well and never had any breathing problems. He was a lifelong non-smoker and he kept no pets. On examination he was beginning to develop clubbing. He was afebrile and looked pale. His pulse was 100/min. Blood pressure was 140/85 mmHg, dropping to 110/70 mmHg on standing. Heart sounds were normal. Coarse crepitations were heard widely, although mainly in the right mid-zone. A spleen tip was palpable. Examination was otherwise normal.

Hb 8.4 g/dl, white cell count $36 \times 10^9/l$ (96% lymphocytes), platelets $240 \times 10^9/l$, MCV 103 fl, Na 144 mmol/l, K 3.7 mmol/l, urea 8.8 mmol/l, creatinine 110 μmol/l, albumin 36 g/l, bilirubin 30 μmol/l, ALT 28 U/l. CXR: fibrotic shadows right mid-zone, hilar lymphadenopathy, no active consolidation.

1. Select the best single diagnosis from each of the groups below:

   a) Chronic myeloid leukaemia
   b) Non-Hodgkin's lymphoma
   c) Multiple myeloma
   d) Chronic lymphocytic leukaemia (CLL)
   e) Bronchoalveolar carcinoma

   f) Pulmonary amyloidosis
   g) Bronchiolitis obliterans
   h) Recurrent community-acquired pneumonia
   i) Secondary bronchiectasis
   j) Proximal bronchial obstruction

   k) Acquired hypogammaglobulinaemia
   l) Bone marrow carcinomatosis
   m) Neutropoenia
   n) Renal loss of immunoglobulins

   o) B12 or folate deficiency
   p) Plasmacytic leukaemia
   q) Cold antibody haemolytic anaemia

r) Warm antibody haemolytic anaemia
s) Aplastic anaemia

Case 4.10

A 44-year-old lady with a 15-year history of primary progressive multiple sclerosis was referred with increasing malaise and dizziness. She had developed an erythematous, markedly swollen area on her left buttock three days previously at the site of occasional intramuscular injections, and she had been commenced on oral antibiotics. However, she felt increasingly hot and unwell, with headache and myalgias as well as increasing pain in her buttock. On examination she had cerebellar speech and signs consistent with a spastic paraparesis with a T10 sensory level. She was peripherally vasodilated, with a blood pressure of 90/60 mmHg. Her pulse rate was 120/min and there was a soft third heart sound. Abdominal examination was normal, although sensation was markedly impaired and she was incontinent of urine. There was an erythematous area on her left buttock, with a central, purplish-brown, non-blanching discoloration. It was non-fluctuant and there was no palpable lymphadenopathy.

1. What is the diagnosis?
   a) Buttock abscess
   b) Cellulitis
   c) Fournier's gangrene
   d) Pyoderma gangrenosum
   e) Necrotizing fasciitis
   f) Ecthyma gangrenosum

2. What is the most important next step?
   a) Surgical referral
   b) Intravenous high-dose antibiotics
   c) Ultrasound of buttock
   d) MRI of buttock
   e) Serial blood cultures from different sites
   f) Wound swab and urgent microscopy

Exam 5

███████

Case 5.1

A 48-year-old cereal farmer presented with increasing breathlessness over one year. Initially intermittent and helped somewhat by a salbutamol inhaler prescribed by his GP, his breathlessness was now nearly continuous. On reflection he thought his symptoms were worse in the evening and when working in the barn. They persisted during the weekend, although had improved during a stay with his son in Manchester. Over the previous three months he had developed a dry cough. There was no relevant previous history and he had never smoked. His examination was normal, apart from slightly quiet breath sounds and occasional wheeze. CXR was normal.

Lung function tests were as follows:

	Predicted	Actual	% predicted
FEV_1	2.87	1.40	48.8
FVC	3.88	2.12	54.1
FEV/FVC (%)	70	66	94.3
RV	2.0	4.1	198
TLC	5.8	6.26	108
KCO	1.44	1.9	133

There was an 8% improvement in FEV_1 with salbutamol.

1. What is the diagnosis?
    a) Silo filler's lung
    b) Farmer's lung
    c) Occupational asthma
    d) Byssinosis
    e) Bagassosis

2. Select the further investigation that would be most informative:
    a) Serial peak flows with documentation of environment
    b) IgE subsets

c) Skin prick testing
d) Bronchial provocation testing
e) High-resolution CT

Case 5.2

A 73-year-old man was referred to the on-call medical team with fever and back pain. He had recently suffered a week-long illness featuring fever, anorexia, frequent foul diarrhoea, and colicky abdominal pain. He thought he had started to recover from this illness when he developed rapidly progressive, severe lower back pain. He smoked 20 cigarettes per day and had suffered an uncomplicated anterior MI four years previously. On examination he was pale and shocked. Temperature was 38.3 °C, pulse rate was 130/min and blood pressure was 90/60 mmHg. His JVP was not raised and heart sounds were normal. There was a large, tense, expansile abdominal mass palpable.

1. What is the diagnosis?
   a) Polyarteritis nodosum
   b) Gastroenteritis and incidental abdominal aortic aneurysm
   c) Inflammatory aortic aneurysm
   d) Mycotic abdominal aortic aneurysm complicating gastroenteritis
   e) Diverticular abscess with direct invasion of aortic wall

Case 5.3

A 10-year-old boy was admitted with dizziness. For the preceding five days he had been febrile, with a sore throat and more recently abdominal pain. On examination he was pale and jaundiced, with an erythematous throat and a palpable spleen.

Hb 8.0 g/dl, white cell count 6.2 × 10⁹/l (neutrophils 60%, lymphocytes 40%), platelets 270 × 10⁹/l, reticulocytes 12%, direct Coombs' test negative, bilirubin 130 μmol/l, no bilirubinuria.

1. What is the cause of his illness?
   a) Congenital haemolytic anaemia with viral URTI
   b) Parvovirus B19 infection
   c) Acute leukaemia
   d) *Mycoplasma pneumonia* infection with cold antibody haemolytic anaemia
   e) Infectious mononucleosis with splenic rupture
   f) Congenital red cell aplasia with viral URTI

Case 5.4

A 48-year-old man presented with a two-hour history of severe crushing chest and epigastric pain with nausea and vomiting. On examination his pulse was 50/min and regular and blood pressure was 130/70 mmHg in both arms. His heart sounds were normal except for a variable intensity of S_1, and his JVP was raised 8 cm, with intermittent cannon waves. Kussmaul's sign was positive. Bibasal crepitations were audible in his chest. He was given 5 mg diamorphine and 40 mg frusemide for the severe pain and clinical heart failure. Fifteen minutes later he was pain-free but feeling faint, with a blood pressure of 70/30 mmHg and pulse of 50/min.

1. Choose the single most likely diagnosis from each of the following groups:

   a) Pulmonary embolism
   b) Aortic dissection
   c) Occlusion of left anterior descending artery
   d) Inferoposterior myocardial infarction
   e) Pancreatitis with early ARDS

   f) Mobitz type 2 heart block
   g) Complete heart block
   h) Slow atrial fibrillation
   i) Reperfusion arrhythmia

   j) Cardiac tamponade
   k) Papillary muscle rupture
   l) Drug-induced vasodilation
   m) Acute ventricular septal defect (VSD)

Case 5.5

An 18-year-old first-year law student was sent up by the college GP because of drowsiness. In hospital he slept for prolonged periods of time and when awoken ate his own plus several other patients' meals. The nurses wanted him to be sent to the psychiatric hospital on account of flirtatious behaviour and, on several occasions, public masturbation. His parents were contacted. They told of similar episodes of abnormal behaviour occurring two and four years previously.

1. What is the diagnosis?
   a) Klüver–Bucy syndrome
   b) Complex partial epilepsy
   c) Klein–Levine syndrome
   d) Schizophrenia

e) Sociopathy
f) Drug abuse
g) Narcolepsy

Case 5.6

A 35-year-old man presented with a long history of non-bloody diarrhoea and abdominal bloating. He had been prone to bouts of diarrhoea since childhood, but symptoms had been worse more recently. He was a well-balanced man with no history of any psychological problems. Examination revealed a midline abdominal scar. No other abnormality was detected.

Full blood count, electrolytes, liver function, ESR, CRP and clotting were all within normal limits. 24-hour stool collection: 500 g (normal: <200 g), pH 5.7, osmolality 430 mosmol/kg (normal: <350 mosmol/kg), Na 85 mM, K 65 mM, fat 23 mmol. Stool weight decreased to 50 g after a three-day fast. OGD was normal. Microscopy of jejunal biopsy was normal. Rectal biopsy showed no melanosis coli. No laxatives were detected in the urine or faeces.

1. Choose the most likely diagnosis from the following:
   a) Irritable bowel syndrome
   b) Jejunal diverticulosis with bacterial overgrowth
   c) Bile salt-induced diarrhoea
   d) Lactase deficiency
   e) Hypogammaglobulinaemia

2. Select the two investigations/management steps that are most likely to help:
   a) Referral for psychological evaluation
   b) Enzymatic assay of brush border of jejunum
   c) Hydrogen breath test
   d) Trial of cholestyramine
   e) IgG subclass determination
   f) Trial of antibiotics
   g) Barium follow-through examination
   h) Reassurance and avoidance of further investigation

Case 5.7

A 24-year-old centre forward sustained a complicated right tibia and fibula fracture following a vicious tackle from behind. The leg was placed in an external fixator. The following day he was placed on flucloxacillin for what appeared to be a wound infection. Three days later, blood tests were sent off prior to a further plating operation. On examination his temperature was 37.6 °C. Apart from the orthopaedic wound, only very mild bilateral flank tenderness was noted. Blood pressure was 130/80 mmHg. He appeared normovolaemic and had no rash.

Hb 12.4 g/dl, white cell count 17.6 × 10⁹/l (55% neutrophils, 35% lymphocytes), Na 135 mmol/l, K 4.8 mmol/l, urea 28.3 mmol/l, creatinine 380 μmol/l. Urine dipstick: blood, protein, and 1+ leucocytes. Ultrasound kidneys: normal size, no evidence of obstruction.

1. What is the most likely diagnosis?
    a) Acute tubular necrosis due to rhabdomyolysis
    b) Renal hypoperfusion due to NSAIDs
    c) Drug-induced acute interstitial nephritis
    d) Fat embolism
    e) Endotoxin-induced renal injury

2. Choose two specific management steps from the following:
    a) Urgent manometry of fascial compartments and fasciotomy
    b) Stop flucloxacillin and NSAIDs
    c) Urinary alkalinization
    d) Start corticosteroids
    e) Change to third-generation cephalosporin and metronidazole
    f) Veno-venous haemofiltration
    g) Debridement of wound site and urgent microscopy/culture
    h) Colloid challenge with CVP monitoring

Case 5.8

A 30-year-old HIV-positive hairdresser presented with gradually increasing fatigue, abdominal pain and pruritus. He had no other past medical history. On examination he was jaundiced with scratch marks, but no xanthelasma, pigmentation or stigmata of chronic liver disease or encephalopathy was apparent. The remainder of the examination was entirely normal.

Full blood count and electrolytes: normal. INR 1.4, bilirubin 57 μmol/l, ALP 580 U/l, ALT 55 U/l.

1. Select the most likely pathology from the following:
    a) Peliosis hepatis
    b) Chronic hepatitis
    c) Metastatic hepatic abscess(es)
    d) Sclerosing cholangitis
    e) Duodenal adenoma
    f) Parasitic obstruction of common bile duct

2. Select the two most likely offending organisms:
    a) *Bartonella quintana*
    b) Epstein–Barr virus

   c) Human herpes virus 8
   d) Cytomegalovirus
   e) HBV
   f) *Helicobacter pylori*
   g) *Streptococcus milleri*
   h) *Opisthorcis sinensis*
   i) *Cryptosporidium parvum*

Case 5.9

A 20-year-old student was admitted through casualty delirious. No history was available. On examination she was febrile at 39.5 °C and sweaty. She looked dry and was tachypnoeic. Her pulse was 110/min and blood pressure was 100/60 mmHg. JVP was not raised and heart sounds were normal. There were scattered bibasal crepitations in the chest. Abdominal examination was normal. No focal neurology was obvious, although examination was difficult due to her lack of co-operation.

Na 144 mmol/l, K 3.0 mmol/l, urea 10.4 mmol/l, creatinine 180 µmol/l, glucose 2.8 mmol/l, ALT 25 U/l, INR 1.3. Blood gases: pH 7.24, pO_2 14.4 kPa, pCO_2 1.8 kPa. CXR: ?occasional interstitial lines.

1. Which single diagnosis best fits this scenario?
   a) Idiosyncratic reaction to ecstasy (MDMA)
   b) Herpes simplex encephalitis
   c) Bacterial meningitis
   d) Salicylate overdose
   e) Paracetamol overdose
   f) Amphetamine overdose
   g) Tricyclic antidepressant overdose

2. From each group below, select the management step that is most important:

   a) Gastric lavage
   b) Blood cultures
   c) Lumbar puncture
   d) Intravenous diazepam

   e) Intravenous N-acetylcysteine
   f) Intravenous aciclovir
   g) Intravenous bicarbonate, potassium and glucose
   h) Intravenous potassium and glucose

   i) Haemodialysis
   j) Broad-spectrum antibiotics

k) Observation only
l) Intravenous fresh-frozen plasma

Case 5.10

An 18-year-old student presented with acute confusion and diarrhoea. She had been well until two days before, gave no history of any infectious contacts, and had undertaken no recent foreign travel. She had eaten similar food to her friends, who had remained well. On examination she looked ill. She was febrile at 38.8 °C, with a subtle but widespread macular erythematous rash. Her pulse was 140/min. Blood pressure was 100/60 mmHg lying down and 70/40 mmHg sitting. An ejection systolic murmur was audible in the aortic area. Her chest was clear. Her abdomen was soft with normal bowel sounds, rectal examination detecting only loose non-bloody stool.

Hb 11.4 g/dl, white cell count 16.7 × 10^9/l, platelets 450 × 10^9/l, Na 138 mmol/l, K 3.8 mmol/l, urea 23.4 mmol/l, creatinine 300 μmol/l. Blood film: normal. Stool, blood and urine cultures were all negative. She was transferred to ICU and resuscitated with colloid and pressor agents.

1. What is the most likely diagnosis?
    a) Acute infective endocarditis
    b) Gastroenteritis complicated by haemolytic uraemic syndrome (HUS)
    c) Rheumatic fever
    d) Scarlet fever
    e) Toxic shock syndrome
    f) Leptospirosis

2. Which of the following regimens is *unlikely* to be helpful?
    a) Intravenous clindamycin
    b) Intravenous flucloxacillin
    c) Intravenous gentamicin
    d) Intravenous vancomycin
    e) Intravenous immunoglobulin

Exam 6

Case 6.1

A 10-year-old boy was referred by his school nurse, who had noticed that his pupils were of unequal size. On examination there was no fatiguability. Adrenaline 1 : 1000 had no effect on pupil size. The following pictures were taken (a) before and (b) after 0.1% pilocarpine administration:

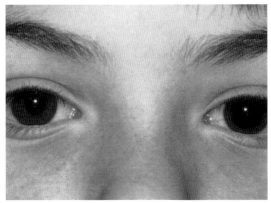

(a)

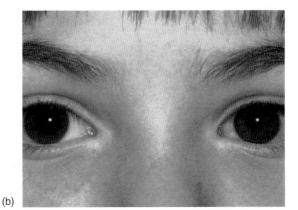

(b)

1. What is the cause of the anisocoria?
   a) Left partial Horner's syndrome
   b) Left Holmes–Adie pupil
   c) Right Holmes–Adie pupil
   d) Right partial Horner's syndrome
   e) Pharmacological mydriasis

Case 6.2

A 32-year-old Brazilian plumber on holiday in the UK for two weeks had been on a five-day alcohol binge at a meeting near Stonehenge. He then travelled up to Scotland, where he suffered a generalized tonic–clonic seizure. He had recovered enough on arrival in hospital to inform the staff of his previous good medical health. The casualty officer arranged a CT scan on account of the following eye abnormality:

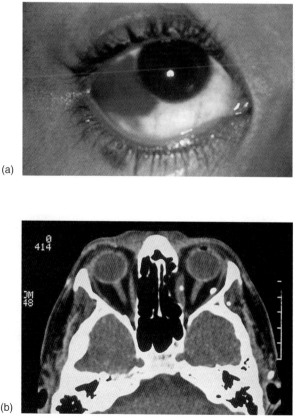

(a)

(b)

1. This shows:
   a) Subhyaloid haemorrhage
   b) Scleritis
   c) Episcleritis
   d) Conjunctival haemorrhage
   e) Battle's sign

2. The CT scan shows:
   a) Fresh contusions
   b) Old contusions
   c) Calcifications
   d) Multiple aneurysms
   e) Multiple metastases
   f) Normal CT scan

3. Select from the following list the two most likely causes for his seizures:
   a) Cerebral contusions
   b) Alcohol withdrawal
   c) Neurocysticercosis
   d) Tuberose sclerosis
   e) Toxoplasmosis
   f) Rubella
   g) Meningiomas

Case 6.3

A 20-year-old student presented with a one-month history of a hoarse voice. Over the preceding year she had been suffering from increasing fatigue, which she ascribed to her studies, shortness of breath and central chest tightness on exertion. She had no cough or haemoptysis and had no past medical or family history. She was taking the contraceptive pill and dieting tablets.

The chest radiograph is shown in the figure at the top of page 45.

1. Which of the following best fits the radiographic appearance?
   a) Bilateral hilar lymphadenopathy and cardiomegaly
   b) Segmental oligaemia and cardiomegaly suggesting pulmonary embolism
   c) Within normal limits
   d) Enlarged left atrium and left atrial appendage
   e) Cardiomegaly, enlarged pulmonary proximal pulmonary vessels, and peripheral oligaemia

2. What is the most likely diagnosis?
   a) Appetite-suppressant-induced pulmonary hypertension with recurrent laryngeal palsy
   b) Grade 1 pulmonary sarcoidosis with infiltration of vocal cords in addition

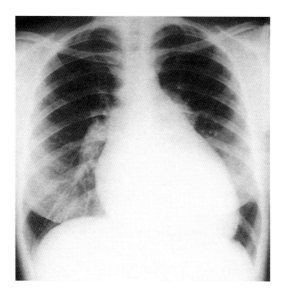

   c) Atrial septal defect
   d) Hodgkin's disease
   e) Cardiomyopathy

Case 6.4

A 20-year-old law student had been becoming more prone to daydreaming during lectures and disinterested in supervisions. She lost contact with her friends. When she had not been seen for two weeks the authorities broke into her room, finding it in an extremely unkempt state. She was lying in a mess of urine and faeces. She was taken to casualty. In casualty she appeared awake but was unable to give any history, except for occasional random yes or no answers. On examination her expression was vacant. She had intact menace reflexes. Pupillary, corneal and gag reflexes were normal. There was no facial asymmetry and no signs of seizure activity. She appeared to resist attempts to assess tone. Reflexes were normal and symmetrical with down-going plantars.

1. Select the two most likely diagnoses from the following list:
   a) Catatonic schizophrenia
   b) Cataplexy
   c) Psychomotor retardation of depression
   d) Drug overdose
   e) Neuroleptic malignant syndrome
   f) Malignant hyperpyrexia
   g) Wilson's disease

2. Select the two most pertinent investigations from the following list:
   a) Serum caeruloplasmin
   b) 24-hour urinary copper levels
   c) Urine drug toxicology screen
   d) CT head scan
   e) HLA testing
   f) Serum CK
   g) EEG

Case 6.5

A 44-year-old lawyer was referred by her firm's doctor because of refractory hypertension. This had first been detected two years before at a routine health check, when the untreated blood pressure had exceeded 160/100 mmHg on three occasions. Since then atenolol 50 mg daily, bendroflumethiazide 2.5 mg daily and amlodipine 10 mg daily, initially singly and latterly together, had been introduced, but the resting supine blood pressure remained 155/105 mmHg. The patient continued to be asymptomatic. She was a non-smoker, she drank around 14 units of wine per week, and her past medical history and family history were unremarkable. Examination in clinic revealed blood pressure of 165/105 mmHg supine and 160/110 mmHg standing. Pulse was 66/min and there was a loud S1. All peripheral pulses were present and examination was otherwise unremarkable. Later fundoscopy showed grade 2 hypertensive retinopathy.

Full blood count was normal. Na 136 mmol/l, K 3.3 mM, urea 6.5 mmol/l, creatinine 114 μmol/l, HCO_3 32 mmol/l. 24-hour urinary VMA and 24-hour urinary free cortisol: normal. CXR: cardiomegaly only.

All medications were stopped for two weeks. After a further week of a high-salt diet, supine 8 a.m. blood tests were as follows: plasma renin activity 8.1 pmol/ml/h (normal: 2.8–4.5), plasma aldosterone concentration 700 pmol/l (normal: 100–450).

1. Select one or more possible underlying diagnoses from the following:
   a) Essential hypertension and continued beta-blocker use
   b) Essential hypertension and continued thiazide use
   c) Renin-secreting tumour
   d) Conn's adenoma
   e) Bartter's syndrome
   f) Bilateral adrenal hyperplasia
   g) Aortic coarctation
   h) Renovascular hypertension
   i) Glucocorticoid-remediable hyperaldosteronism

Among other investigations, a renal angiogram was later performed; this is shown in the following figure.

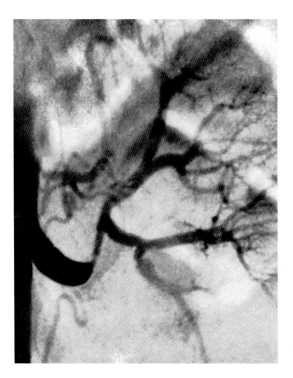

2. Which of the following is most consistent with this appearance?
    a) No renal cause for hypertension
    b) Atherosclerotic renal artery stenosis
    c) Fibromuscular dysplasia (FMD)
    d) Tumour blush from secretory renal tumour
    e) Duplex kidney

Case 6.6

A 44-year-old HIV-positive antiques dealer presented with a two-month history of progressive shortness of breath, weight loss and vague pains underneath his sternum. He felt tired. His past medical history was unremarkable except for an attack of herpes zoster four years earlier. He did not smoke, and he drank alcohol only occasionally. He had no family history of note. He had been otherwise well.

Hb 9.5 g/dl, white cell count 3.5 × 10⁹/l (80% neutrophils), urea 43 mmol/l, creatinine 78 μmol/l, CK 130 mmol/l. CXR: enlarged heart, clear lung fields. The chest radiograph and part of the ECG rhythm strip are shown in the following figures.

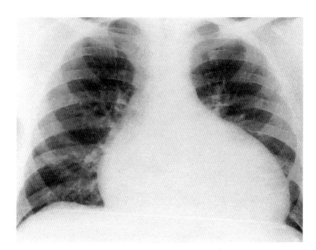

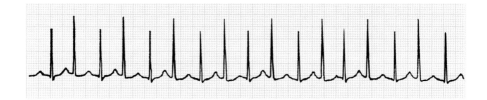

1. Give the most likely underlying diagnosis from the following:
   a) *Mycobacterium tuberculosis* infection
   b) Coxsackie virus infection
   c) Tertiary *Treponema pallidum* infection
   d) Ischaemic heart disease
   e) Autoimmune myocarditis
   f) HIV-induced cardiomyopathy

Case 6.7

A 54-year-old man presented with a six-month history of progressive clumsiness and difficulty in performing fine tasks with his right hand. He had no pain. Apart from a chronic cough he was well. Past medical history was unremarkable. He was adopted and did not know his family history. He smoked 40 cigarettes per day. General examination, higher mental function and cranial nerve examination were all normal. The intrinsic muscles of his right hand were slightly wasted, and occasional fasciculations were seen both here and in his left biceps and triceps. Intrinsic hand muscle strength was weak, more so on the right. Reflexes and co-ordination were normal, and there was no sensory deficit to pain, temperature, vibration or proprioception testing. Lower limb and sphincter examinations were entirely normal.

Full blood count, electrolytes, liver function tests, clotting, ESR, CRP, CXR, CT head and MRI of cervical spine were all normal. TPHA, VDRL, ANA, anti-dsDNA and rheumatoid factor were all negative.

1. Give the three most important differential diagnoses from the following list:
   a) Inclusion body myositis
   b) Multifocal motor neuropathy with conduction block
   c) Hereditary motor and sensory neuropathy (HMSN) type 1a
   d) HMSN type 1b
   e) HMSN type II
   f) Motor neuron disease (MND)
   g) Cervical radiculopathy
   h) Kennedy's syndrome
   i) Paraneoplastic motor neuropathy
   j) AIDP
   k) Porphyria
   l) Lead poisoning

Case 6.8

A 47-year-old man presented with gradually increasing weakness of his right leg over a period of 24 hours. Over the subsequent 24 hours his other leg also became weak and he developed a headache. While in the ambulance he had a generalized tonic–clonic convulsion, which was terminated with diazepam. In his past history he had been warfarinized for six months following a DVT and had been diagnosed five years ago with irritable bowel syndrome. He now took no medications. General examination was normal. Higher mental function was normal except for slight drowsiness. Pupillary reactions, visual fields and eye movements were all normal.

The fundal appearance is shown below:

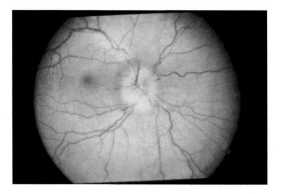

1. Which description best fits the fundal appearance?
   a) Diabetic retinopathy
   b) Central retinal vein occlusion
   c) Central retinal artery occlusion
   d) Papilloedema
   e) Retinal vasculitis

   The reminder of the cranial nerve exam was normal. Upper limbs were normal. Hip flexion was grade 4/5 bilaterally. Ankle plantar flexion and dorsiflexion was 3/5 on the right and 4/5 on the left. Knee jerks were normal but six beats of clonus were elicitable at the right ankle and five at the left. Both plantars were up-going.

2. What is the most likely diagnosis?
   a) Anterior spinal vein and central retinal vein thromboses
   b) Anterior spinal artery and central retinal artery infarcts
   c) Hypertensive encephalopathy and spinal cord infarct
   d) Spinal cord and cerebral abscesses
   e) Sagittal sinus thrombosis
   f) Poorly controlled diabetes
   g) Bifrontal infarcts
   h) CNS vasculitis
   i) Sarcoidosis

3. From the following, select one investigation to carry out:
   a) Lumbar puncture with opening pressure
   b) Blood glucose
   c) CT head with contrast
   d) MRI spine
   e) ESR
   f) ANA
   g) Serum ACE
   h) CXR

Case 6.9

A man presents with a novel neurological syndrome. The extended family are traced and examined:

1. What is the likely mode of inheritance?
   a) Autosomal dominant
   b) Autosomal recessive
   c) Maternal genomic imprinting
   d) Mitochondrial transmission
   e) Paternal genomic imprinting
   f) X-linked dominant

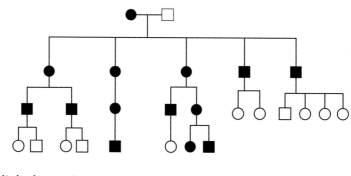

g) X-linked recessive
h) Y-linked

Case 6.10

A 55-year-old man presented with increasingly severe frontal headaches, which were worse on bending over or coughing. He also complained of nausea and vomiting. He had developed a cough and brought up fresh blood on several occasions. His past medical history was unremarkable. He smoked 20 cigarettes per day and drank 30 units of alcohol per week.

Full blood count and electrolytes were normal. CXR: multiple nodular shadows and enlarged right hilum.

He was commenced on dexamethasone and maintenance intravenous fluids for presumed raised intracranial pressure. The following morning his Na was 155 mmol/l.

1. What is the likely cause of the rise in serum sodium?
   a) Nephrogenic diabetes insipidus
   b) Cranial diabetes insipidus
   c) SIADH of cranial origin
   d) SIADH of pulmonary origin
   e) Severe hyperglycaemia
   f) Adrenal haemorrhage
   g) Inappropriate fluid regimen

Exam 7

Case 7.1

An 18-year-old university student called out his GP because of severe generalized non-pleuritic chest pain. Earlier that day his wisdom teeth had been removed under general anaesthetic with succinylcholine (suxamethonium) and propofol induction and isoflurane maintenance as a day case. The operation had been successful as far as he knew.

1. What is the diagnosis?
    a) MI
    b) Succinylcholine myalgia
    c) Neuroleptic malignant syndrome
    d) Succinylcholinesterase deficiency
    e) Malignant hyperpyrexia
    f) Hypertrophic obstructive cardiomyopathy (HOCM)

Case 7.2

A 14-year-old boy presented to casualty with a small ulcer on his leg. This had begun as a small, pruritic, indurated nodule that was due, he thought, to a scratch. However, over a three-week period it had spread and begun to ulcerate, despite the use of tetracycline and metronidazole from his GP. He had emigrated recently from Uganda to join his father in the UK. On examination he looked and felt well. The ulcer was 4 × 3 cm and appeared superficial, with overhanging edges. There was no pain, tenderness or lymphadenopathy.

1. What is the most likely diagnosis?
    a) Buruli ulcer
    b) Pyoderma gangrenosum
    c) Tropical ulcer
    d) Endemic syphilis
    e) Yaws
    f) Pinta

Case 7.3

A 47-year-old man gradually became increasingly lethargic over a three-week period, with nausea, vomiting and headaches, before eventually presenting to hospital with diplopia. He was febrile and drowsy. His facial appearance (looking to the right) is shown here:

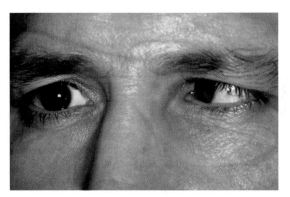

1. What does this picture show?
   a) Right III nerve palsy
   b) Left III nerve palsy
   c) Right IV nerve palsy
   d) Left IV nerve palsy
   e) Right VI nerve palsy
   f) Left VI nerve palsy

   Examination was otherwise normal. Na 127 mmol/l. CT normal. CSF: 200 lymphocytes, protein 1.2 g/l, glucose 1.0 mmol/l (blood 5.5 mmol/l), Gram stain negative.

2. What is the most likely cause of his drowsiness?
   a) Fungal meningitis, e.g. coccidioidomycosis
   b) *Mycoplasma*-associated aseptic meningoencephalitis
   c) Tuberculous meningitis
   d) Carcinomatous meningitis
   e) Sarcoidosis
   f) Partially treated bacterial meningitis
   g) Syphilis
   h) Herpes simplex encephalitis

3. Select two possible explanations from the following for the sodium level:
   a) SIADH
   b) Adrenal failure

c) Water intoxication
d) Artefactual

Case 7.4

A 38-year-old alcoholic presented with a six-week history of increasing shortness of breath. He had no chest pain, cough, haemoptysis or sputum production. On examination he smelled of alcohol, was confused, and had four spider naevi on his chest. There was no asterixis.

This was one of the patient's hands:

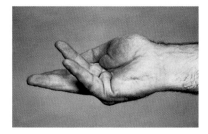

1. What abnormality does he have in his hands?
   a) Combined median and ulnar nerve compression palsies
   b) Dupuytren's contracture
   c) Volkmann's ischaemic contracture

2. The JVP waveform and phonocardiogram (below) show:
   a) Giant a waves
   b) Giant v waves
   c) Normal waveform
   d) Dichrotic notch
   e) Canon waves

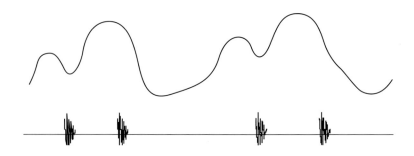

His pulse was 120/min and blood pressure 120/50 mmHg. On auscultation he had a gallop rhythm and bilateral basal crepitations. A 2-cm tender liver edge was palpable. His ankles were swollen. Neurological examination was normal except for slight ataxia and absent ankle jerks.

Na 136 mmol/l, K 4.6 mmol/l, urea 7.6 mmol/l, creatinine 130 μmol/l, chloride 92 mmol/l, glucose 4.5 mmol/l, bicarbonate 16 mmol/l, osmolality 330 mosmol/kg.

3. The electrolytes show:
   a) Normal anion gap
   b) Raised anion gap

4. What is the diagnosis?
   a) Wet beriberi
   b) Alcoholic cardiomyopathy
   c) Methanol poisoning

5. How would you confirm the diagnosis?
   a) B12 levels
   b) Red cell transketolase activity
   c) Cardiac biopsy
   d) Echocardiogram
   e) Examine urine for oxalate crystals
   f) Blood methanol levels

Case 7.5

A 56-year-old lady was refered to the pain clinic on account of uncontrollable back pain. History-taking was difficult because she was still in a lot of pain and the history given was colourful in content. She said she had suffered with a more or less constant gnawing ache in her lower thoracic spine for two years. Nothing seemed to make it better. She had taken paracetamol, NSAIDs, codeine and morphine and was using a TENS machine. Physiotherapists and occupational therapists had been involved, to no avail, and she was consuming liberal amounts of alcohol to try and afford some sort of relief. MRI of her entire spine had revealed widespread degenerative disease, although this was mainly in cervical and thoracic areas and of moderate degree. There appeared to be no area of obvious cord or root compression. In the past she had dislocated a shoulder during a fight when she was 18, and when she was 24 she 'slipped a lumbar disc'. This was managed conservatively, with success. On examination movement and upper abdominal compression seemed to make the pain worse. Apart from nine spider naevi, the examination was normal.

Hb 10.2 g/dl, white cell count 5.5 × 10⁹/l, platelets 340 × 10⁹/l, MCV 105 fl, Na 144 mmol/l, K 4.4 mmol/l, urea 2.4 mmol/l, creatinine 60 μmol/l, glucose 9.5 mmol/l, calcium 2.2 mmol/l, phosphate 1.1 mmol/l, albumin 32 g/l, ALT 50 U/l, bilirubin 24 μmol/l, ALP 80 U/l.

1. What is the diagnosis?
   a) Duodenal ulcer
   b) Locally invasive oesophageal carcinoma complicating pernicious anaemia
   c) Uncontrolled diabetes with hepatic steatosis
   d) Myelopathy not seen on MRI
   e) Chronic pancreatitis

2. From each of the four groups below select the investigation/treatment that is *not* likely to be useful:

   a) 75-g oral glucose tolerance test
   b) ERCP
   c) Trial of long-acting epidural anaesthetic injections

   d) Plain abdominal radiography
   e) Pentagastrin stimulation test
   f) Secretin stimulation test

   g) Faecal elastase determination
   h) Faecal occult blood determination
   i) Serum vitamin B12 determination

   j) Trial of pancreatic enzyme supplements
   k) OGD and biopsy
   l) Vitamin D determination

Case 7.6

A 45-year-old bartender presented with acute haematemesis and melaena. She felt slightly dizzy when standing up but was otherwise well. Her past medical history consisted of otitis externa and an open cholecystectomy. She recalled having rigors after her surgery and needing a prolonged course of antibiotics. She smoked 10 cigarettes per day but claimed to be teetotal. She had no family history and took no drugs. On examination there were no stigmata of chronic liver disease. She was not encephalopathic but she was pale. Blood pressure was 120/80 mmHg, dropping to 90/60 mmHg on standing. Pulse was 120/min and heart sounds were normal. Her liver was not palpable but a 4-cm spleen was felt. There was no detectable ascites.

Hb 8.5 g/dl, white cell count 5×10^9/l, platelets 440×10^9/l. Electrolytes, liver function tests and clotting were all normal. OGD: bleeding varices. Wedged hepatic venous pressure: normal.

1. What is the most likely diagnosis?
   a) Hepatitis C cirrhosis
   b) Alcoholic cirrhosis

c) Primary biliary cirrhosis
d) Presinusoidal portal hypertension secondary to biliary sepsis
e) Splenic vein thrombosis
f) Chronic non-alcoholic steatohepatitis

Case 7.7

A 36-year-old man presented in status epilepticus. He responded to diazepam and on recovery said he had been suffering with headaches for the last week. On examination he was thin, with axillary, cervical and inguinal lymphadenopathy.

1. What abnormality is seen on his leg (shown below)?
   a) Erythema nodosum
   b) Mycosis fungoides
   c) Granuloma annulare
   d) Kaposi's sarcoma
   e) Syphilitic gumma

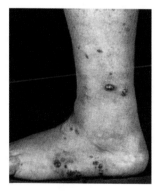

The remainder of a general examination was normal. He had no meningism.

2. What does his fundal photograph (following figure) show?
   a) CMV retinitis
   b) Candle-wax dripping
   c) Miliary tuberculosis
   d) Normal fundus
   e) Syphilis

He had a left homonymous hemianopia. The remainder of the cranial nerve examination was normal. He had mild, left-sided pyramidal weakness, particularly in the upper limb, with corresponding brisk reflexes and an up-going left plantar. Sensation and co-ordination were normal.

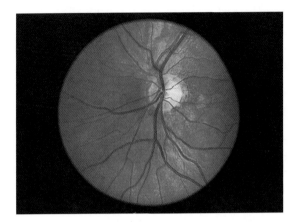

The patient's T2-weighted MRIs looked as follows:

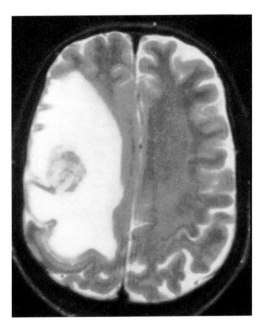

3. What are the two most likely diagnoses for this appearance?
    a) Lymphoma
    b) Sarcoid granuloma
    c) Syphilitic gumma
    d) Tuberculoma
    e) Toxoplasmosis

  f) Cryptococcoma
  g) Bacterial abscess
  h) Progressive multifocal leukoencephalopathy (PML)

4. What is your first management strategy?
  a) Intravenous penicillin
  b) Intravenous penicillin plus corticosteroids
  c) High-dose intravenous methylprednisolone
  d) Therapeutic trial of anti-tuberculous therapy
  e) Therapeutic trial of antifungal therapy
  f) Therapeutic trial of anti-toxoplasma drugs
  g) Biopsy lesion
  h) Lumbar puncture
  i) Cefotaxime and gentamicin and metronidazole

Case 7.8

A 55-year-old businessman presented with a one-year history of weakness and clumsiness. Initially he noticed that he was tripping over his right foot and then found it difficult climbing stairs. He also found gardening much more difficult and was unable to lift a spade. He complained of intermittent paraesthesiae in his hands. In his past medical history he was hypertensive with a raised cholesterol, and he had contracted gonorrhoea once on a business trip. He took aspirin, simvastatin and atenolol. He smoked five cigars per day and drank half a bottle of wine with his evening meal. On examination he was tanned, with a blood pressure of 120/80 mmHg and no postural drop. Cardiovascular, respiratory and abdominal examinations were normal. Higher mental function and cranial nerve examination were normal. His right triceps, left biceps and interossei in both hands were wasted. Occasional fasciculations were seen. There was a corresponding weakness. All upper limb reflexes were normal. Tone was increased in his lower limbs. There was no evident wasting or fasciculation. There was weakness of plantar and dorsiflexion in both feet, more so on the right. Both knee jerks were brisk, and there were five beats of clonus at each ankle. Both plantars were up-going. There were no cerebellar signs, and a full sensory examination was normal.

1. Select three investigations from the following list that you would carry out:
  a) MRI head
  b) MRI cervical spine
  c) TPHA and VDRL
  d) CK
  e) PMP22 gene testing
  f) EMG
  g) Lumbar puncture
  h) Nerve biopsy
  i) Muscle biopsy

Case 7.9

A 24-year-old nurse presented with recurrent attacks of sweating and dizziness, particularly on waking. She had no previous history and examination was normal. Blood samples were obtained during a period of dizziness. Full blood count, electrolytes, calcium, phosphate and liver function tests were normal. Blood glucose 1.1 mmol/l, plasma C-peptide 15 nmol/l (normal fasting: <0.4 nmol/l).

1. Which further step should be taken first?
   a) 72-hour fast
   b) Plasma and urine sulphonylurea determination
   c) Abdominal ultrasonography
   d) Locker search for insulin
   e) Short synacthen test

Case 7.10

A 14-year-old boy was referred on account of his failing academic performance at school and disruptive influence. His mother said that he was very conscientious in many ways, often to extremes, checking his bag ten times in the morning to make sure all his schoolbooks were packed and washing his hands dozens of times after going to the toilet. However, in class he would sometimes repeatedly shake his head or raise his hand in the air even if he did not want to ask a question. At other times he would grunt or squeal out loud. The teachers became increasingly angry when these grunts started to sound very like obscenities. When told to shut up he would often repeat the teacher's words. Worse still, he would occasionally make obscene gestures at them.

1. What is the diagnosis?
   a) Obsessive-compulsive disorder
   b) Gilbert's syndrome
   c) Gilles de la Tourette's syndrome
   d) Bad upbringing
   e) Wilson's disease
   f) Klein–Levine syndrome

Exam 8

███████████

Case 8.1

A 19-year-old student is referred from casualty for overnight observation. She had become increasingly distressed during the course of a friend's party. She was known to be seeing a psychiatrist, but no other history was available. On examination she was anxious and sweating profusely.

Saturation 100% on air, temperature 39.5 °C, respiratory rate 40/min, pulse 140/min, blood pressure 110/65 mmHg, heart sounds normal. Chest clear. Abdomen soft. No focal neurology, although assessment was difficult as she was holding herself very stiffly. No meningism. ECG and CXR both normal.

Hb 12.8 g/dl, white cell count 9.8×10^9/l, Na 138 mmol/l, K 5.2 mmol/l, urea 7.4 mmol/l, creatinine 132 μmol/l

1. Select the two most likely diagnoses from the following list:
    a) Idiosyncratic reaction to ecstasy (MDMA)
    b) Malignant hyperpyrexia
    c) Tetany
    d) Tetanus
    e) Poisoning from drugs cut with strychnine
    f) Drug withdrawal
    g) Rhabdomyolysis
    h) Catatonia
    i) Neuroleptic malignant syndrome

Case 8.2

A 47-year-old businesswoman underwent surgery to debulk an ovarian neoplasm. Postoperatively she bled extensively despite good surgical haemostasis.

Hb 7.2 g/dl, platelets 160×10^9/l, PT 14 s (normal: 10–12 s), APTT 40 s (normal: 26–32 s) correcting with normal plasma, thrombin time 45 s (normal: 10–12 s), fibrinogen 0.01 g/l (normal: 1.5–4.0 g/l), FDPs 300 mg/l (normal: <10 mg/l).

1. What is the best diagnosis?
    a) Disseminated intravascular coagulation
    b) Acquired haemophilia

   c) Von Willebrand's disease type 2
   d) Hyperfibrinolysis
   e) Antiphospholipid syndrome

2. Which of the following treatments is *unlikely* to help?
   a) Tranexamic acid
   b) Fresh-frozen plasma
   c) Aminocaproic acid
   d) Desmopressin (DDAVP)
   e) Aprotinin

Case 8.3

A 27-year-old lady presented to casualty with persistent bleeding following extraction of a painful, carious second left upper premolar tooth. She was known to have a prolapsing mitral valve, and three months previously she had suffered a miscarriage. Otherwise her past medical and family history were unremarkable. Examination was normal.

   Hb 13.2 g/dl, platelets 240×10^9/l. Film: normal platelet appearance. PT 13 s (normal: 10–12 s), APTT 40 s (normal: 32–37 s), TT 12 s (normal: 11–12 s). Bleeding time prolonged to >10 min. Clot solubility test normal. Von Willebrand antigen level normal. Ristocetin-induced platelet aggregation normal. Normal platelet aggregation to ADP but impaired aggregation to collagen. Electrolytes and liver function normal.

1. What is the most likely diagnosis?
   a) Drug-induced platelet dysfunction
   b) Haemophilia
   c) Storage pool disease
   d) Antiphospholipid syndrome
   e) Type 2 von Willebrand's disease

Case 8.4

A 45-year-old man was admitted because of falls. He had been fit throughout his life but over the previous six months had suffered from increasingly severe postural presyncope and had become more constipated. He had no past medical history. On examination his skin was dry. His pulse was 70/min and regular and did not vary with posture, unlike his blood pressure, which dropped from 140/70 mmHg to 70/30 mmHg. He was not dehydrated or pale. On neurological examination cranial nerves were normal. He had no wasting or fasciculations. Tone and power were normal. Pain and temperature sensation were decreased in his feet. Reflexes were all normal, with down-going plantars. Full blood count, electrolytes and CXR were all normal. ECG showed no sinus arrhythmia.

1. Which of the following is the most likely diagnosis?
   a) Thoracic cord lesion
   b) Conus lesion
   c) Small-fibre peripheral neuropathy
   d) Large-fibre peripheral neuropathy

Case 8.5

A 40-year-old lady developed right upper quadrant pain two weeks after a fall. She felt nauseated but had not vomited, and she was passing dark urine and pale stools. Her past medical and family histories were unremarkable. On examination she was overweight and jaundiced. Her temperature was 38.1 °C, blood pressure was 110/60 mmHg and pulse was 100/min. Heart sounds were normal and her chest was clear. Her right upper quadrant was tender, with 4-cm smooth hepatomegaly and a soft hepatic bruit. No splenomegaly or ascites were detected.

Na 136 mmol/l, K 3.6 mmol/l, urea 3.6 mmol/l, creatinine 108 µmol/l, bilirubin 280 µmol/l, ALT 50 U/l, AST 122 U/l, ALP 320 U/l, GGT 430 U/l, Hb 11.4 g/dl, white cell count 16.2×10^9/l, platelets 280×10^9/l, INR 1.3. CXR: clear lung fields, fractured ribs. Ultrasound: homogeneous hepatomegaly. Several gallstones in gallbladder. Normal biliary tree.

1. What is the most likely diagnosis?
   a) Acute cholecystitis
   b) Ascending cholangitis
   c) Infected hepatic haematoma
   d) *Streptococcus milleri* liver abscess
   e) Alcohol-induced hepatitis
   f) Non-alcoholic steatohepatitis

2. Select one test from the following to confirm your diagnosis:
   a) Liver ultrasonography
   b) Abdominal X-ray
   c) ^{99m}Tc-HIDA scintiscan
   d) ERCP
   e) Liver biopsy
   f) Surgery

Case 8.6

A 30-year-old HIV-positive man developed a severe pneumonic illness. Bronchoscopic lavage confirmed pneumocystis infection. He recovered with high-dose co-trimoxazole and steroids and was maintained on zidovudine (AZT), lamivudine, indinavir and co-trimoxazole. He was reasonably well for 18 months, before beginning to lose considerable weight and becoming more lethargic. He began to have night sweats. A full examination revealed no specific pathology, although his temperature was 37.9 °C.

Hb 8.6 g/dl, white cell count 3.2×10^9/l, platelets 130×10^9/l. Film: normochromic with anaemia, lymphopenia, thrombocytopenia. Electrolytes: normal. ALT 65 U/l, ALP 297 U/l, albumin 30 g/l, bilirubin 8 μmol/l. Saturation on air after exercise 100%. CXR: normal. Blood, urine and faeces culture: negative. DEAFF test on blood and urine: negative. CD4 count 30/mm^3.

1. Which two diagnoses from the following should be pursued first?
    a) Disseminated cryptococcosis
    b) Disseminated *Mycobacterium avium intracellulare* infection
    c) Drug fever
    d) AIDS-associated generalized wasting syndrome
    e) CMV infection
    f) Lymphoma
    g) Occult Kaposi's sarcoma
    h) Parvovirus B19 infection

2. Suggest from the following the next two steps to be taken:
    a) Bone marrow aspirate and trephine
    b) CT abdomen
    c) Change drug regimen
    d) PCR of peripheral blood for CMV
    e) Bronchoscopy and lavage
    f) Trial of anabolic steroids
    g) CT brain with contrast

Case 8.7

A 60-year-old lady with a five-year history of type II diabetes was found to be hyperkalaemic. She had felt quite well, except for occasional angina, arthritis and 'irritable bowel syndrome'. In her past medical history she had had bilateral cataract extractions three years previously and laser therapy to her left eye two months before. Her medications consisted of gliclazide, simvastatin, indomethacin and GTN.

Na 135 mmol/l, K 5.9 mmol/l, urea 9.3 mmol/l, creatinine 130 μmol/l, albumin 36 g/l, calcium 2.3 mmol/l, phosphate 1.3 mmol/l, chloride 114 mmol/l, bicarbonate 14 mmol/l. Short synacthen test: normal cortisol response but recumbent aldosterone levels low.

1. What is the most likely diagnosis?
    a) Early adrenal failure
    b) Allergic tubulointerstitial nephritis due to indomethacin
    c) Gordon's syndrome

d) Type 1 renal tubular acidosis (RTA)
e) Type 4 RTA
f) Excess gastrointestinal bicarbonate loss

2. Which of the following would be most consistent with your diagnosis?
   a) Arterial blood pH 7.2, urinary pH 6.3, low daily acid secretion
   b) Arterial blood pH 7.26, urinary pH 5.3, low daily acid secretion
   c) Arterial blood pH 7.34, high daily acid secretion, negative urine anion gap
   d) Arterial blood pH 7.2, urinary pH 5.3, normal daily acid secretion
   e) Arterial blood pH 7.2, urinary pH 5.3, high plasma renin level

Case 8.8

A 24-year-old launderette assistant presented with a two-week history of headaches. She decided to seek medical attention when she developed double vision. On direct questioning, she would occasionally lose her vision bending over. She was, however, otherwise well. Systems enquiry was unremarkable, except for long-standing period irregularity. She did not think she was pregnant. Her past medical history was unremarkable. On examination she was overweight with nicotine-stained fingers. General examination and higher mental function were normal.

Below is a view of her fundus:

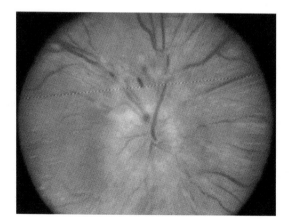

1. Which of the following descriptions is likely to best fit this lady?
   a) Fields were constricted, with detectable enlargement of both blind spots. Acuity 6/6

b) Fields were constricted, with detectable enlargement of both blind spots. Acuity 6/60
c) Fields were normal. Acuity 6/6
d) Fields were normal. Acuity 6/60

On examination she had bilateral sixth nerve palsies. The remainder of the neurological examination was normal.

2. What is the most likely diagnosis?
   a) Idiopathic intracranial hypertension
   b) Pontine tumour, with secondary hydrocephalus
   c) Normal-pressure hydrocephalus
   d) Bilateral optic neuritis and brainstem demyelination

Case 8.9

An 18-year-old student decided to take up rowing, with some success, winning his first five-mile race. That night he awoke with marked weakness of his limbs, such that it was difficult to reach the phone. Sensation remained entirely normal. However, by the time his GP arrived the student was better. Six weeks later, after his next race, a similar weakness developed overnight. When seen in hospital 12 hours later, his weakness had once again subsided. He had no past medical history of note and took no drugs. He was unaware of his family history as he was adopted. Examination was entirely normal.

Full blood count and electrolytes were normal. CK was normal. Urine dipstick was normal. ECG was normal.

1. Give the two most likely differential diagnoses from the following list:
   a) Hypokalaemic periodic paralysis
   b) Traumatic cervical myelopathy
   c) Myasthenia gravis
   d) Acute inflammatory demyelinating polyneuropathy
   e) Chronic inflammatory demyelinating polyneuropathy
   f) Poliomyelitis
   g) Hypokalaemic weakness
   h) Guillain–Barré syndrome

2. Select the two investigations from the following list that confirm most easily these two potential diagnoses:
   a) Thyroid function tests
   b) Anti-acetylcholine receptor antibody
   c) EMG
   d) Muscle biopsy
   e) Serum potassium during attack
   f) Ischaemic muscle forearm test

g) Nerve conduction studies
h) Tensilon test

Case 8.10

A 30-year-old man presented with a one-hour history of crushing central chest pain with no radiation. He felt nauseated and was sweaty. In the past he had suffered intermittent severe burning pains and tingling in his hands and feet, particularly during a change of temperature or on exercise, and had been noted by his GP to suffer from Raynaud's phenomenon. He did not smoke and he drank alcohol only occasionally. He knew his cholesterol was not raised, but he did not know whether he had any family history of heart disease as he was adopted. On examination he was in pain. No rheumatological abnormalities were apparent, but patchy skin lesions were noted on the scrotum and trunk, as shown below:

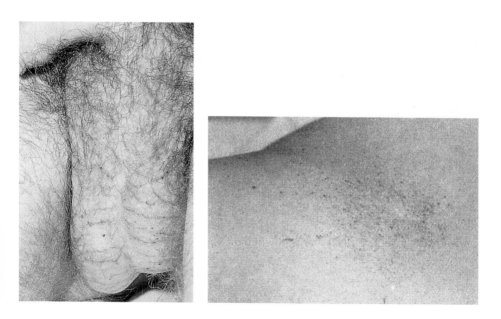

His pulse was 100/min, blood pressure was 150/100 mmHg, JVP was not raised, heart sounds were normal, apex beat was undisplaced, and chest was clear. There was no organomegaly.

1. What are the two likely diagnoses?
   a) MI
   b) Urticaria pigmentosum

c) Ehlers–Danlos syndrome type IV
d) Fabry's disease
e) SLE
f) Porphyria cutanea tarda
g) Scleroderma
h) Aortic dissection
i) Oesophagitis
j) Pseudoxanthoma elasticum

Exam 9

Case 9.1

A 19-year-old labourer was admitted as an emergency after 48 hours of abdominal pain. He felt nauseated but had a normal bowel habit. He was otherwise fit and well and had no infectious contacts. He had never been abroad. On examination he was febrile at 38.6 °C, with a tender abdomen. He displayed guarding and rebound in the right iliac fossa. Rectal examination was normal apart from some right-sided tenderness. Abdominal and erect chest radiographs were normal. At operation a normal appendix was removed. The terminal ileum was inflamed and the ileocaecal nodes were markedly enlarged, with adjacent hyperaemia of the mesentery. His abdominal pain and fever were still present 72 hours postoperatively, prompting a referral to the medical registrar.

1. Which of the following underlying diagnosis is most likely?
    a) Crohn's disease
    b) *Yersinia* infection
    c) Ileal tuberculosis
    d) Small bowel lymphoma
    e) Whipple's disease

Case 9.2

A 44-year-old man spilt soap into his right eye during washing. Whilst blinded temporarily in that eye, he discovered he was blind in the other. His visual fields are shown below:

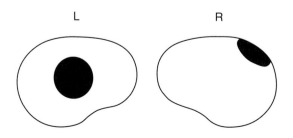

1. On the basis of the information in this chart, one would predict that pupillary testing would:
   a) Be normal
   b) Reveal a left afferent pupillary defect
   c) Reveal a right afferent pupillary defect
   d) Reveal a left pupil unreactive to light but reactive to accommodation
   e) Reveal a right pupil unreactive to light but reactive to accommodation

   The left optic disc was slightly pale. The remainder of the examination was normal.

2. What is the diagnosis?
   a) Anterior chiasmal compression
   b) Optic nerve compression
   c) Retrobulbar neuritis
   d) Optic neuritis

Case 9.3

A 22-year-old unemployed man presented with a three-month history of progressive weakness and tingling feet. He commented on occasional abdominal pain but otherwise his past medical and family history were unremarkable. On examination he was slovenly and appeared drunk. He had normal visual acuity.

This is a picture of his retina:

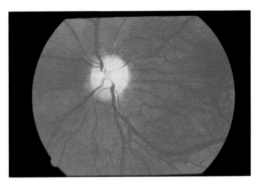

1. What does his fundal appearance show?
   a) Optic disc pallor
   b) Cherry red spot
   c) Retinitis pigmentosa
   d) Angioid streaks

   He was globally weak, proximally more so than distally. There was no fatiguability. Reflexes were normal in the upper limbs, but knee jerks were obtainable only with reinforcement and ankle jerks were absent. Plantars were down-going.

He had slight intention tremor and past pointing and an ataxic gait, although weakness complicated this assessment. Apart from some erythematous acneiform spots around his mouth and nose, the remainder of the examination was normal.

2. Which of the following is the most likely diagnosis?
   a) Fabry's disease
   b) Spinocerebellar ataxia type 1
   c) Spinocerebellar ataxia type 2
   d) Spinocerebellar ataxia type 3
   e) Pseudoxanthoma elasticum
   f) Organic solvent toxicity
   g) Tay–Sach's disease
   h) Thiamine deficiency
   i) Wernicke–Korsakoff syndrome

Case 9.4

A 30-year-old man presented with a two-year history of progressive numbness, which had begun in his buttocks and gradually spread down the back of his legs into the soles of his feet. His legs were also weak. More recently he had become impotent and incontinent of both faeces and urine. He had no past medical history. On examination his neck appeared normal, with no bruits and no pain on movement. Buttocks and calves were wasted, with weakness bilaterally of hip extension and ankle dorsi and plantar flexion. Knee jerks were present, but ankle jerks and plantar responses were absent. A sensory deficit was evident, extending from the anus down the back of the legs on to the soles. The anal sphincter was lax.

1. Where anatomically is/are the lesion(s)?
   a) Bilateral sacral plexus lesion
   b) Conus medullaris
   c) Cauda equina
   d) Sciatic nerves
   e) Distal spinal cord

2. Suggest from the following a likely diagnosis:
   a) Sarcoidosis
   b) Multiple sclerosis
   c) Central disc prolapse
   d) Tumour or cyst
   e) Degenerative spondylolisthesis

Case 9.5

A 23-year-old woman presented six weeks postpartum with a rash, malaise and lymphadenopathy. She had immigrated from Ghana during her pregnancy. She said she had been treated in Africa shortly before falling pregnant for a painless ulcerating papule on her vulva associated with painless groin lymphadenopathy.

VDRL, TPHA and IgG FTA-Abs were all positive. HIV ELISA was negative.

1. Choose one or more interpretations of her serology from the following:
    a) Secondary syphilis following failure to eradicate primary infection before conception
    b) Reinfection with syphilis after initial eradication of primary infection before conception
    c) Adequately treated primary syphilis pre-conception, now false-positive VDRL with rash unrelated to syphilis
    d) Childhood exposure to endemic syphilis, chancroid pre-conception, current viral illness
    e) HIV co-infection with syphilis pre-conception, with syphilis adequately treated
    f) Postpartum HIV infection with previously adequately treated syphilis

2. Which one of the following tests on the mother would be *least* useful?
    a) VDRL titre
    b) Dark-field microscopy of lymph node aspirate
    c) Western blot of peripheral blood
    d) HIV RNA PCR
    e) HIV DNA PCR

3. Which of the following tests on the baby would be useful?
    a) HIV ELISA
    b) IgM FTA-Abs
    c) IgG FTA-Abs
    d) VDRL
    e) HIV ELISA delayed to six months

Case 9.6

A 42-year-old woman developed a sore throat and cough. She felt lethargic, she had lost her appetite, and her knees and ankles ached. She sought medical attention when she passed blood in her urine some days later. On examination her throat was erythematous and enlarged lymph nodes were palpable in the upper cervical chain. There was a rash on both legs, extending to the buttocks, a detail of which is shown in the figure at the top of page 73.

Her knees and ankles were tender to touch and slightly swollen.

1. What is the best diagnosis?
    a) Infectious mononucleosis complicated by thrombocytopoenia
    b) Henoch–Schönlein purpura (HSP)
    c) Post-streptococcal glomerulonephritis

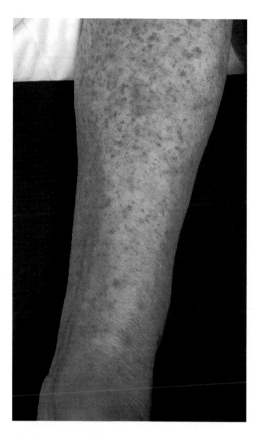

d) IgA nephropathy/Berger's disease
e) Acute leukaemia with bone marrow failure

2. Which single diagnostic test would you select?
   a) Renal biopsy
   b) Electrolytes
   c) Urine microscopy
   d) Biopsy skin lesion
   e) Bone marrow aspirate and trephine
   f) Lymph node biopsy
   g) Monospot test
   h) Antistreptolysin O titre (ASOT)/anti-DNAse B/anti-hyaluronidase

Case 9.7

A 28-year-old man complained of increasing nocturia over a period of several weeks. He suffered from bipolar depression and had been maintained on lithium for the previous three years.

Na 123 mmol/l, K 2.8 mmol/l, urea 1.7 mmol/l, creatinine 45 μmol/l, Li 0.5 mmol/l, glucose 3.6 mmol/l, cholesterol 2.2 mmol/l, triglycerides 0.7 mmol/l. Immunoglobulins: normal. Urine osmolality 50 mosmol/kg.

1. What is the diagnosis?
   a) Dipsogenic diabetes insipidus
   b) Nephrogenic diabetes insipidus
   c) Cranial diabetes insipidus
   d) SIADH
   e) Addison's disease

Case 9.8

A 38-year-old lady presented with pain in her fingers, particularly at night. She was a single mother with one child. She had had one miscarriage. She also suffered bad heartburn and since her teens had been prone to Raynaud's phenomenon. She took no medication, did not smoke or drink, and had no relevant family history. The appearance of her face is shown below:

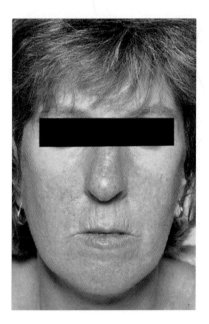

A diagnosis was made. After 12 years of follow-up she complained of shortness of breath. On re-examination, she was tachypnoeic and centrally cyanosed. Her chest was clear on auscultation, but a loud second heart sound was noted. Her chest radiograph showed no signs consistent with pulmonary fibrosis. Her ECG is shown in the following figure.

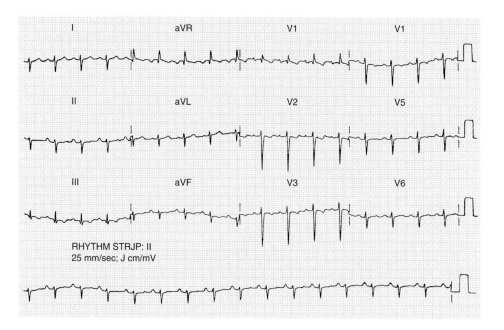

RHYTHM STRJP: II
25 mm/sec; J cm/mV

A V/Q scan was abnormal but reported as being more in keeping with intrinsic lung pathology than pulmonary emboli.

1. What was the diagnosis at presentation?
   a) Hereditary haemorrhagic telangiectasiae
   b) Mixed connective tissue disease
   c) Limited cutaneous scleroderma
   d) Diffuse cutaneous scleroderma
   e) Antiphospholipid syndrome
   f) SLE

2. What was the cause of her breathlessness?
   a) Pulmonary hypertension
   b) Pericardial effusion
   c) Pulmonary fibrosis
   d) Fibrosing alveolitis
   e) Pulmonary AV shunting

Case 9.9

A 44-year-old teacher was referred to the respiratory out-patient department with chest pain. This had been present for nearly one year, intermittent at first but now nearly continuous. The pain was aching and central, sometimes worse lying flat and sometimes worse on inspiration. Two episodes of pleurisy had been treated with antibiotics. She smoked 20 cigarettes per day and had progressive shortness of breath, particularly when lying flat. She was asthmatic as a child and suffered with Raynaud's phenomenon.

1. Which two of the following are most consistent with this pattern of shortness of breath?
   a) Deficient abdominal musculature
   b) Hepatic cirrhosis with pulmonary AV shunting
   c) Bilateral diaphragmatic weakness
   d) Cardiomyopathy
   e) Pulmonary sarcoidosis

On examination she was apyrexial. A pericardial rub was audible but her chest was clear. No other abnormality was detected.

Hb 10.5 g/dl, white cell count 12.2×10^9/l, ESR 99 mm/h. Electrolytes and liver function tests were normal. Rheumatoid factor was negative.

The chest radiograph was reported to show slight cardiomegaly, bilaterally raised hemidiaphragms and some bibasal atelectasis. Lung function tests revealed a restrictive defect but with a normal KCO.

2. What is the most likely diagnosis?
   a) Myasthenia gravis
   b) Ischaemic heart disease and Dressler's syndrome
   c) SLE and shrinking lung syndrome
   d) Carcinomatous pericarditis
   e) Polymyositis

3. Select from the following the two investigations most likely to lead to the diagnosis:
   a) Anti-acetylcholine receptor antibodies
   b) Anti-dsDNA antibody
   c) Anti-Jo antibody
   d) High-resolution CT chest
   e) Fluoroscopic study of chest
   f) Tensilon test
   g) Flow-volume loop
   h) Aspiration and microscopy of pleural fluid
   i) Echocardiography

Case 9.10

A 16-year-old shop assistant complained that over the previous few months she kept on falling over. She said that suddenly her legs would just buckle. She did not lose consciousness and there were no jerking movements. The falls seemed to occur whenever she laughed or got angry. Similarly, when emotional her head had, on occasion, dropped forward and her jaw dropped down. These periods of weakness had lasted one minute at longest. She was otherwise well, with no past medical or family history of note. A full examination was normal.

1. What is the diagnosis?
   a) Catatonia
   b) Benign postural vertigo
   c) Negative myoclonus
   d) Narcolepsy
   e) Atonic seizures

2. Select a treatment from the following:
   a) Imipramine
   b) Cinnarizine
   c) Carbamazepine
   d) Amphetamines
   e) Sodium valproate

Exam 10

Case 10.1

A 52-year-old baker presented to clinic with increasing shortness of breath over two months. He was a lifelong smoker of 20 cigarettes per day, but until now he had enjoyed good health. In contrast, his father, brother and uncle had all died of stomach cancer. Clinically he had a large left pleural effusion, which was confirmed on CXR. Aspiration revealed a white fluid. There was no clear supernatant after centrifugation. No cholesterol crystals could be detected.

1. What is the nature of the pleural fluid?
    a) Chyle
    b) Stomach contents
    c) Empyema
    d) Pseudochyle
    e) Liquefied necrosis

2. What is the most likely underlying cause?
    a) Tuberculosis
    b) Yellow nail syndrome
    c) Lung cancer
    d) Hiatus hernia
    e) Lymphoma
    f) Lymphangioleiomyomatosis

Case 10.2

A 26-year-old secretary presented with a six-month history of increasing breathlessness and non-productive cough. She had no orthopnoea or chest pain. She smoked 20 cigarettes per day. In her past medical history she had bad cradle cap as an infant and seborrhoeic eczema as a child. She developed a limp aged seven, which settled with conservative treatment, and pain in her right upper arm aged 13 and 17, again settling spontaneously. She suffered intermittent otitis externa. Examination revealed decreased chest expansion with diffuse fine inspiratory crepitations. Apart from eczema in her inguinal and axillary areas, examination was normal. Lung function tests showed a mild restrictive pattern with a reduced diffusion capacity. Full blood count, electrolytes and coagulation studies were all normal.

1. Which of the following diagnoses explains the clinical findings most fully?
   a) Lymphangioleiomyomatosis
   b) Hypogammaglobulinaemia
   c) Langerhans' cell histiocytosis
   d) Letterer–Siwe disease
   e) Sarcoidosis

2. Which of the following is the most appropriate initial investigation?
   a) Bone marrow aspirate
   b) High-resolution chest CT
   c) Bronchoalveolar lavage
   d) Serum ACE level
   e) Biopsy of unaffected skin
   f) Plasma electrophoresis

Case 10.3

An 18-year-old gardener presented with a six-month history of urinary frequency and nocturia. He commented that he had occasionally passed blood after a chest cold. Past medical history was unremarkable, although his brother was deaf and he thought some 'eye trouble' ran in the family. Examination was normal. He proceeded to have a CXR, IVP and cystoscopy, all of which were normal. He was therefore discharged from clinic, but he re-presented three years later in end-stage renal failure. Anti-GBM antibody and ANCA were both negative. He was commenced on haemodialysis, but after only three months an autologous kidney, HLA-matched in three out of four loci, was transplanted without complication. The transplanted kidney was working well until six months postoperatively, when the patient became oliguric with a rising creatinine. Cyclosporin levels were normal. A renal biopsy showed a crescentic glomerulonephritis. Anti-GBM antibody was positive and ANCA was negative.

1. Which of the following is the most likely underlying cause of his initial end-stage renal failure?
   a) Microscopic polyangiitis
   b) Wegener's granulomatosis
   c) Goodpasture's syndrome with false-negative anti-GBM antibody
   d) Alport's syndrome
   e) Diabetic nephropathy
   f) AA amyloidosis due to chronic bronchiectasis
   g) IgA nephropathy
   h) Primary hyperparathyroidism
   i) Pendred's syndrome
   j) Churg–Strauss syndrome

2. From the same list, select the most important alternative diagnosis

3. Why did the transplant fail?
   a) Alloimmunization to missing antigen
   b) Recurrent glomerulonephritis
   c) Graft rejection
   d) Persisting metabolic insult
   e) Accelerated amyloid deposition due to immunosuppression

Case 10.4

A nine-year-old boy had been unwell with high fevers for one week. His GP had prescribed amoxicillin for conjunctivitis on day three, but with no effect. On examination he was febrile at 39.2 °C, with enlarged cervical lymph nodes. His oral cavity, lips and pharynx were erythematous. There was a morbilliform rash covering the trunk and limbs, and his fingers were markedly swollen. The following week he became breathless.

1. What is the most likely diagnosis?
   a) Kawasaki disease
   b) Rheumatic fever
   c) Scarlet fever
   d) Stevens–Johnson syndrome
   e) Acute lymphoblastic leukaemia

2. Which two of the following treatments should he have had initially?
   a) Aspirin
   b) Intravenous penicillin
   c) Parenteral hydrocortisone
   d) High-dose erythromycin
   e) Induction chemotherapy
   f) Plasma exchange
   g) High-dose gammaglobulin
   h) Oral ciprofloxacin
   i) Cessation of all medication
   j) Intravenous vancomycin

Case 10.5

A 45-year-old insurance salesman presented with a nine-month history of weight loss and pale, foul-smelling diarrhoea. He had lost weight and been troubled by mouth ulcers, but he had suffered no abdominal pain. He had had a chronically blocked nose and intermittent sinusitis for as long as he could remember, and he said that winter colds would always go to his chest. He smoked 10 cigarettes per day and drank alcohol occasionally. He habitually spent part of the year in Portugal. On examination he was thin and pale. An aphthous ulcer was present under his tongue. Examination was otherwise normal.

Hb 9.2 g/dl, MCV 105 fl, serum B12 100 ng/l, red cell folate 90 μg/l, Fe 8 μmol/l, calcium 2.3 mmol/l, phosphate 1.1 mmol/l, ALP 130 U/l, INR 1.2. 24-hour faecal fat excretion: 50 mmol/day. Hot stool sample: microscopy and culture negative. CXR: normal. Barium follow-through: multiple small lymphoid nodules.

1. Give two likely diagnoses from the following:
   a) Ciliary dyskinesia
   b) Giardiasis
   c) Bacterial overgrowth
   d) Small bowel T-cell lymphoma
   e) Coeliac disease
   f) IgA deficiency
   g) Crohn's disease
   h) Whipple's disease
   i) HIV infection

2. Which one of the following is most likely to help as part of the treatment regime?
   a) Metronidazole
   b) Prednisolone
   c) Highly active anti-retroviral therapy (HAART)
   d) Erythromycin
   e) Ciprofloxacin
   f) Surgery

Case 10.6

A 48-year-old man presented with a two-hour history of crushing central chest pain. His ECG is shown in the figure at the top of page 82.

Alteplase (rt-PA) was infused, but over the next hour he became progressively more hypotensive. On examination he had cool peripheries. The pulse was 130/min and regular. Blood pressure was 80/50 mmHg. His JVP was not raised. A mid to late systolic murmur loudest at the lower left sternal edge was audible with a loud S3. The patient said that a murmur had been noticed at an insurance medical four years previously. A Swann–Ganz catheter was floated. RA 5 mmHg, RV 60/10 mmHg, PAWP 15 mmHg, cardiac index 7.2 l/min/m² (normal 2.5–4.0 l/min/m²).

1. What is the diagnosis?
   a) Ruptured ventricular septum
   b) Acute mitral regurgitation

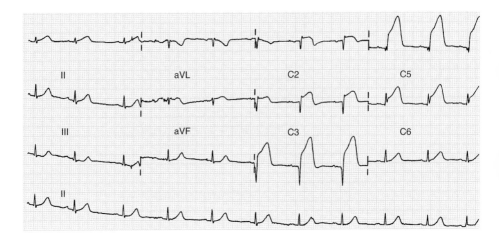

c) Extension of infarct
d) Ruptured ventricular free wall

2. Which of the following is true with regard to this man's further management?
   a) Noradrenaline is likely to reduce the cardiac output
   b) Intra-aortic balloon pumping (IABP) is contraindicated
   c) Surgery should be delayed for several weeks to allow fibrous tissue to form
   d) Medical therapy alone results in 30% in-hospital mortality

Case 10.7

A 70-year-old woman presented with a three-week history of malaise, fevers and a rash on her legs. She had previously been a keen hillwalker but had given up seven years previously on account of angina. She was then found to have a stenotic aortic bicuspid valve and diffuse moderate triple vessel disease. She underwent Bjork–Shiley aortic valve replacement five years previously. This helped her angina initially, although it had been becoming more severe of late, necessitating further diagnostic angiography five weeks before. She had had no operations since the valve replacement, and she had not visited the dentist recently. Her sister had type 2 diabetes. Her medication was warfarin, atenolol, slow-release nifedipine and slow-release nitrate. She previously smoked 40 cigarettes per day but gave up after surgery. She drank alcohol occasionally.

She was afebrile. There was no lymphadenopathy, and hand examination was normal. The pulse rate was 60/min and regular. Blood pressure was 180/110 mmHg. Her JVP was not raised, and fundoscopy was normal. Crisp mechanical heart sounds were audible, together with a soft ejection systolic murmur. A left carotid bruit was heard. The apex beat was undisplaced and of normal character. Good volume peripheral pulses were palpable. There was no organomegaly. The appearance of her legs is shown here:

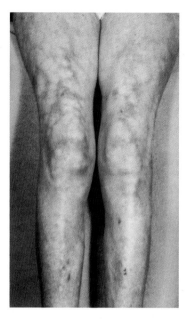

Hb 10.4 g/dl, white cell count 13.6 × 10⁹/l (3% eosinophils), Na 138 mmol/l, K 4.4 mmol/l, urea 26.7 mmol/l, creatinine 310 μmol/l, ALT 123 U/l, albumin 36 g/l, globulin 78 g/l. Three sets of blood cultures: no growth. Transthoracic echocardiogram: normal. ANA, ANCA, anti-dsDNA, anticardiolipin antibodies all negative. Urine dipstick: protein ++, red cells +. Urine microscopy: red cells, occasional hyaline cast. CXR: normal.

1. Which diagnosis most completely explains the findings above?
   a) Non-infective thrombotic (marantic) endocarditis
   b) Cryoglobulinaemia
   c) Churg–Strauss syndrome
   d) Cholesterol emboli
   e) Infective endocarditis
   f) Microscopic polyangiitis

2. Which of the following is most likely to give a definitive diagnosis?
   a) Renal biopsy
   b) PCR of blood for fastidious organisms
   c) Transoesophageal echocardiography
   d) Bone marrow aspirate and cytology
   e) CT imaging of chest and abdomen

Case 10.8

A 40-year-old lady presented with a two-month history of progressive difficulty hanging out her washing and climbing out of a chair. In her past medical history she suffered from Raynaud's phenomenon and heartburn. She took occasional antacids but nothing else. On examination she had marked weakness of her neck and proximal muscles. There was no fatiguability. Reflexes and sensation were normal. Indeed, the remainder of the examination was normal.

Hb 10.4 g/dl, MCV 85 fl, white cell count $6.6 \times 10^9/l$ (neutrophils 70%, lymphocytes 30%), platelets $180 \times 10^9/l$, ESR 60 mm/h. Electrolytes, liver function tests, TSH, calcium, phosphate, CXR and V/Q scan: normal. Rheumatoid factor and ANA: negative.

Over the next eight weeks she became increasingly breathless.

1. Select the most likely underlying diagnosis from the following list:
   a) Limb girdle dystrophy
   b) Polymyositis
   c) Dermatomyositis
   d) Metabolic myopathy
   e) Polymyalgia rheumatica (PMR)
   f) SLE
   g) Scleroderma

2. Which investigation would confirm the diagnosis?
   a) Temporal artery biopsy
   b) Muscle biopsy
   c) Creatinine kinase
   d) ESR
   e) Serum immunoglobulins

Case 10.9

A 74-year-old man arrived in the quick-access clinic having suddenly lost the vision in his right eye 48 hours previously. Prior to this event he had been fit and well, with no past medical history of note. On examination visual acuity was 6/60 in the right eye and 6/6 in the left eye. There was no field defect and no macular sparing. There was a right afferent pupillary defect. The right optic disc appeared swollen but pale, with a flame-shaped haemorrhage at 6 o'clock. Eye movements were full and non-painful. The remainder of the neurological examination and a full general examination were normal.

1. What is the diagnosis?
   a) Retrobulbar neuritis
   b) Pituitary apoplexy
   c) Anterior ischaemic optic neuropathy (AION)

    d) Optic neuritis

    e) Papilloedema

2. Choose one investigation from the following:

    a) ESR

    b) MRI brain and optic nerves

    c) Lumbar puncture with opening pressure measurement

    d) ANA

Case 10.10

A 68-year-old man developed sudden severe left-sided abdominal pain while straining to pass a stool. He had a long tendency towards constipation. He related that on several previous occasions he had developed a similar pain for a few hours, the passage of diarrhoea and flatus heralding the resolution of the pain. He was a type II diabetic controlled with glibenclamide and he was trying, unsuccessfully, to lose weight. On examination he was in pain but afebrile. His abdomen was distended, particularly on the left side, which was tender and tympanitic, with very active bowel sounds. Rectal examination was normal. Apart from background diabetic retinopathy and impaired vibration sense in his feet, the remainder of the examination was normal. Erect CXR was normal. The abdominal radiograph is shown below:

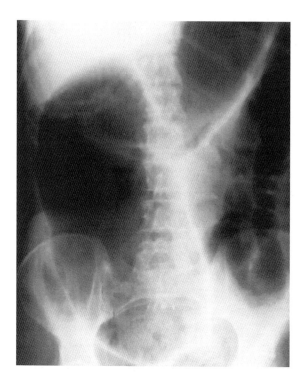

1. What is the diagnosis?
   a) Intussusception
   b) Diabetic autonomic neuropathy
   c) Sigmoid volvulus
   d) Obstructing sigmoid carcinoma
   e) Ischaemic colitis
   f) Sigmoid diverticular disease
   g) Colonic pseudo-obstruction (Ogilvie's syndrome)

Exam 11

Case 11.1

A 74-year-old retired Welsh coal miner presented with a six-month history of pain in his ankles, knees and wrists, for which he been treated by his GP with NSAIDs. He had suffered a short-lived attack of pleurisy five years previously, but otherwise he had been well. The appearance of his hands and his chest radiograph are shown in the following figures.

The rheumatoid factor titre was 1/64. An isotope bone scintigram showed symmetrical increased uptake in the distal femora, tibiae and fibulae.

1. Select the two most likely diagnoses from the following:
   a) Caplan's syndrome
   b) Small-cell lung carcinoma
   c) Pulmonary rheumatoid nodule
   d) Hypertrophic pulmonary osteoarthropathy (HPOA)
   e) Non-small-cell lung carcinoma
   f) Rheumatoid arthritis

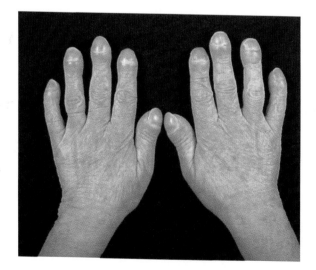

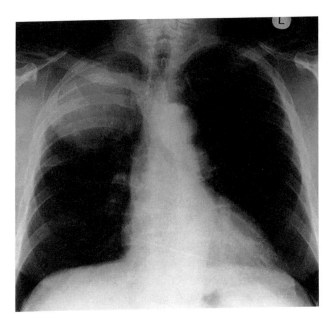

   g) PTHrP-mediated hypercalcaemia
   h) Pseudoclubbing and osteitis fibrosa cystica
   i) Osteoarthritis

Case 11.2

A 35-year-old male nurse, previously well and taking no medication, was noted at an insurance medical to have a serum potassium level of 2.6 mmol/l. Questioned more closely, he confessed to feeling constantly fatigued and to having a fondness for salty foods. His blood pressure was 120/70 mmHg supine and 120/80 mmHg standing. The rest of the examination was normal.

More detailed investigations are shown below:

Serum: Na 140 mmol/l, K 2.7 mmol/l, urea 4.6 mmol/l, Cr 92 μmol/l, Mg 0.54 mmol/l, HCO 31 mmol/l, osmolality 282 mosmol/kg. Renin 6.5 pmol/ml/h (normal: 2.8–4.5 pmol/ml/h), aldosterone 470 pmol/l (normal: 100–450 pmol/l)

Urine: Na 82 mmol/l, K 61 mmol/l, osmolality 221 mosmol/kg. 24-h urine: Ca 0.5 mmol (normal: 3–7 mmol), PO₄ 22.6 mmol (normal: 16–32 mmol), free cortisol 180 nmol (normal: 0–280 nmol).

1. Which of the following are the two most likely diagnoses?
   a) Hypokalaemic periodic paralysis
   b) Bartter's syndrome

c) Cyclical Cushing's syndrome
d) Covert frusemide abuse
e) Familial hypocalciuric hypercalcaemia
f) Gitelman's syndrome
g) Excess liquorice ingestion
h) Laxative abuse
i) Type 2 renal tubular acidosis
j) Conn's adenoma

Case 11.3

A 45-year-old businessman taking ibuprofen for tennis elbow presented faint with melaena. Endoscopy revealed a duodenal ulcer, which was injected with adrenaline and sclerosant. He was transfused with four units of blood and placed on esomeprazole. His recovery was uneventful until his re-presentation at one week with epistaxis and extensive petechiae.

Hb 9.6 g/dl, white cell count 6.3×10^9/l, platelets 12×10^9/l. Film: thrombocytopenia. Bone marrow: increase in megakaryocytes.

1. What is the most likely diagnosis?
   a) Idiopathic thrombocytopenia
   b) Transfusion-related purpura/thrombocytopenia
   c) Drug-induced thrombocytopenia
   d) Transfusion-acquired CMV infection
   e) Splenic vein thrombosis

2. Select the next step from the following:
   a) Fibrin-degradation products
   b) Antiplatelet A1 antibodies
   c) Abdominal ultrasonography with Doppler traces
   d) Blood and urine PCR for CMV
   e) Cessation of proton pump inhibitor
   f) Steroid therapy

Case 11.4

A 54-year-old man presented with increasing breathlessness over three months. He had no chest pain, cough, sputum production or fever. He gave a 20-year history of secondary progressive multiple sclerosis with dysarthria and a spastic paraparesis. He was wheelchair-bound and performed intermittent self-catheterization. He was taking baclofen for painful lower limb flexor spasms. On examination he had multiple ecchymoses on his arms and legs. The appearance of his mouth is shown below:

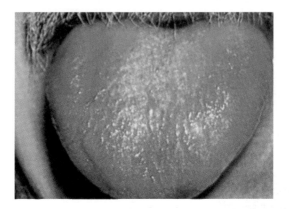

There was obvious facial oedema. The JVP was raised at 8 cm, and there was a fourth heart sound. The pulse rate was 80/min and blood pressure was 130/80 mmHg. Bibasal crepitations were audible in his chest. A 3-cm liver edge was palpable, and there was gross pitting oedema to the waist. He had dysarthric speech, bilateral optic atrophy, bilateral internuclear ophthalmoplegia, and a spastic paraparesis with a sensory level at T11.

Urine dipstick: protein ++++, blood +. Urine microscopy: occasional red blood cells, no white cells, no organisms.

1. What is the most likely diagnosis?
    a) AL amyloidosis
    b) NSAID-induced membranous glomerulonephritis
    c) AA amyloidosis
    d) Renal failure due to recurrent pyelonephritis
    e) Transthyretin-associated amyloidosis

2. Which two of the following will lead most simply to the definitive diagnosis?
    a) Rectal biopsy
    b) Liver biopsy
    c) 24-hour urine protein
    d) Plasma electrolytes
    e) IVP
    f) Urine electrophoresis
    g) Renal biopsy
    h) Endomyocardial biopsy

Case 11.5

A 64-year-old woman presented with a four-week history of weight loss, increasing clumsiness and unsteadiness of gait. She had no other symptoms and no past medical or family history. She was teetotal. On examination she displayed bilateral past pointing, dysdiadochokinesis and truncal ataxia. A full examination was otherwise normal. Full blood count, electrolytes, CXR and ECG were all normal.

1. Her CT scan (below) shows:
    a) Displaced fourth ventricle
    b) Abnormal signal intensity in cerebellum
    c) Normal CT scan
    d) Atrophy of vermis

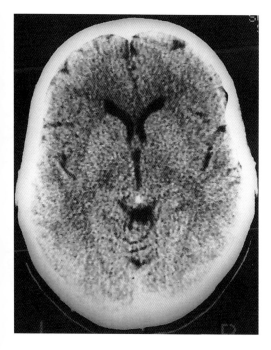
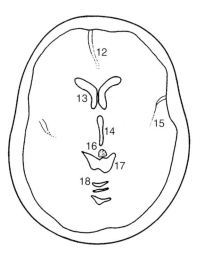

2. What is the most likely diagnosis?
    a) Cerebellar metastases
    b) Medulloblastoma
    c) Paraneoplastic cerebellar degeneration
    d) Hypothyroidism
    e) Alcoholism
    f) Wernicke's encephalopathy

3. Select four investigations from the following that you would carry out:
    a) Anti-Purkinje cell (paraneoplastic) antibodies
    b) Liver function tests
    c) Thiamine levels
    d) Thyroid function tests
    e) Mammogram

f) Pelvic ultrasound
g) CSF analysis
h) Biopsy of cerebellar lesion

Case 11.6

A 16-year-old girl presented with progressive fatigue and swollen ankles. She had a good appetite but was losing weight. She had no nausea, vomiting or abdominal pain, but she had had loose stools for many months. There was no blood in her stools but they were sometimes pale. She had no past medical or family history and, until this problem, had been well. She took no drugs. On examination both legs were swollen. Her hands and face also appeared slightly swollen. Height and secondary sexual characteristics were normal. There was no rash or lymphadenopathy. Her JVP was not raised, blood pressure was 110/70 mmHg and pulse was 80/min. Her heart sounds were normal and apex beat undisplaced and of normal character. Respiratory and abdominal examinations were normal.

Hb 11.5 g/dl, white cell count $4.5 \times 10^9/l$ (90% neutrophils, 5% monocytes, 5% lymphocytes), platelets $340 \times 10^9/l$. Na 137 mmol/l, K 3.6 mmol/l, urea 4.1 mmol/l, creatinine 77 μmol/l, albumin 22 g/l, calcium 2.2 mmol/l, phosphate 0.8 mmol/l, ALP 150 U/l, ALT 22 U/l, CRP < 2 mg/l. IgG 3.8 g/l, IgM 0.2 g/l, IgA 0.3 g/l. Urine dipstick: normal. CXR and small-bowel follow-through: normal.

She was placed on a gluten-free diet, with no benefit.

1. What is the most likely diagnosis?
   a) Small-bowel lymphoma
   b) Small-bowel tuberculosis
   c) Heavy-chain disease
   d) Primary lymphangiectasia
   e) Hypogammaglobulinaemia
   f) Abetalipoproteinaemia
   g) Amyloidosis

2. Which one of the following would be part of the treatment?
   a) Low-fat diet enriched with long-chain triglycerides
   b) Low-fat diet enriched with medium-chain triglycerides
   c) Regular intravenous immunoglobulin
   d) Albumin infusion
   e) Corticosteroids
   f) Prophylactic antibiotics

Case 11.7

A 78-year-old man presented with recurrent falls. Past medical history was unremarkable except for a nasal polypectomy and prostate resection. His brother had coeliac disease. Full blood count, electrolytes, liver function, CT head, carotid Doppler and echocardiogram were all normal. However, his 24-hour tape revealed runs of 2 : 1 block associated with his symptoms of dizziness. A VVI pacemaker was therefore fitted. At follow-up clinic he was still feeling faint, particularly when starting to walk, and he felt that his heart was missing beats. On examination he was suntanned with bilateral arcus and cataracts, a pulse rate of 70/min, a variable S_1 and a clear chest. The JVP during symptoms is sketched below:

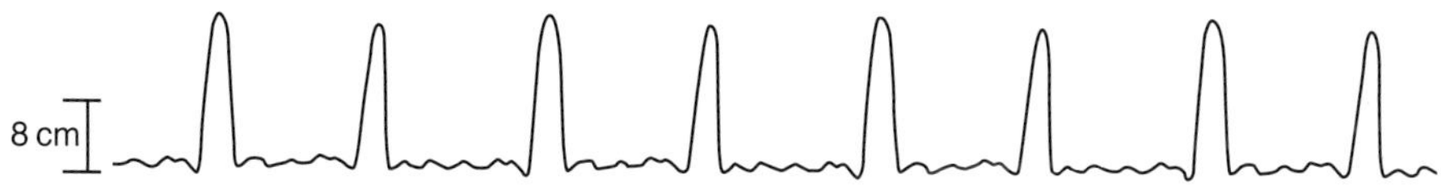

8 cm

1. What is the diagnosis?
    a) Pacemaker lead fracture
    b) Pacemaker malfunction with junctional rhythm
    c) Pacemaker malfunction with complete heart block
    d) Pacemaker syndrome
    e) Tachy/brady syndrome

2. What is the treatment?
    a) Increase the pacing threshold
    b) Set the output rate to the same as the trigger rate
    c) Replace the ventricular lead
    d) Insert an atrial lead and institute atrial pacing
    e) Insert an atrial lead and institute dual-chamber pacing

Case 11.8

A 30-year-old woman underwent cardiac catheterization. The results are shown below:

	Pressure (mmHg)	O$_2$ saturation (%)
SVC		57
RA	12/0	84
RV	40/8	87
PA	37/200	83
PCWP	9	
LV	128/5	98
Aorta	125/70	

1. Which electrocardiographic feature would be most likely in association with the above findings?
   a) Anterior ST elevation
   b) RSR' in lead V1 with right axis deviation
   c) RSR' in lead V1 with left axis deviation
   d) P mitrale
   e) Left bundle branch block
   f) QRS alternans

2. Which two of the following are most consistent with the catheter data?
   a) Reversed splitting of S2
   b) Digital clubbing
   c) Clubbing of fingers but not toes
   d) Pulmonary ejection systolic murmur
   e) Subsequent cerebral infarct following a deep vein thrombosis
   f) Mid-diastolic murmur loudest at the apex
   g) Double right heart border on chest radiograph
   h) Single, loud second heart sound
   i) Dilated left ventricle on two-dimensional echocardiography

Case 11.9

A 24-year-old lady was referred up with weight gain and acne. She had given birth to a healthy baby boy 18 months previously. She had no other symptoms, had no previous medical history, and was taking no medications. On examination she was centrally obese with thin skin and striae. Her blood pressure was 160/100 mmHg. Visual fields were full. No other abnormality was found. Before her follow-up clinic was due, she presented as an emergency with sudden-onset left-sided headache, nausea and double vision. On examination she was drowsy. Pulse was 90/min. Blood pressure was 120/80 mmHg. There was no neck stiffness. Fields were full and fundi were normal. This is a picture of a patient with similar eye signs:

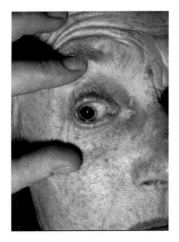

The remainder of the examination was normal.

1. What is the most likely diagnosis?
   a) Idiopathic intracranial hypertension
   b) Pituitary apoplexy
   c) Addison's disease
   d) Intracranial aneurysm
   e) Sheehan's syndrome

2. Choose one investigation from the following:
   a) Urgent CT or MRI pituitary
   b) Cerebral angiogram
   c) Lumbar puncture
   d) Synacthen test

Case 11.10

A known alcoholic was admitted following a focal motor seizure beginning in his right arm, which became secondarily generalized. On examination he was comatose but with no focal neurological deficit. He was tachypnoeic and tachycardic, with a blood pressure of 100/60 mmHg. His JVP was visible at 3 cm, with a normal waveform. His heart sounds were normal but bibasal crepitations were present. It was thought most likely to be a 'rum fit', but as he did not smell of alcohol a CT was requested. This was normal.

Hb 15.6 g/dl, white cell count 12.4 × 10⁹/l, platelets 380 × 10⁹/l, INR 1.2, Na 144 mmol/l, K 5.9 mmol/l, urea 14.5 mmol/l, creatinine 201 μmol/l, calcium 1.8 mmol/l, phosphate 1.1 mmol/l, pO_2 13.5 kPa, pCO_2 2.2 kPa, pH 7.0. CXR: upper lobe diversion and Kerley B lines. Slight cardiomegaly. ECG: right bundle branch block. Urine dipstick: protein +. He was transferred to ICU and given general supportive care.

1. What is the diagnosis?
   a) Methanol poisoning
   b) Tricyclic antidepressant overdose
   c) Ethylene glycol poisoning
   d) Rhabdomyolysis due to recurrent seizures
   e) Acute pancreatitis

2. Select one further investigation from the following:
   a) Urine lipase
   b) Inspection of urine sample under UV light
   c) Urine myoglobin determination
   d) Serum and urine toxicology screen
   e) Addition of Ehrlich's aldehyde to urine specimen

   f) Serum ethylene glycol level
   g) Serum alcohol level

3. Select one treatment from the following:
   a) 1.4% sodium bicarbonate infusion
   b) Ethanol infusion
   c) Forced diuresis
   d) Mechanical hyperventilation
   e) Supportive care only
   f) N-acetyl cysteine infusion

Exam 12

Case 12.1

A 76-year-old lady was sent in by her GP from a nursing home with shortness of breath and cough productive of six cups of mucoid sputum daily. This had been ever present for five months despite admissions two and three months earlier for courses of intravenous antibiotics. She was a lifelong non-smoker with an unremarkable past medical history. Her CXR on readmission is shown below:

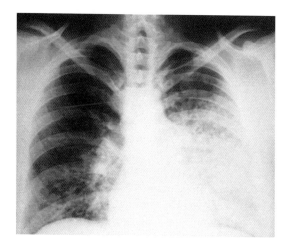

Fibre-optic bronchoscopy was normal. The mucoid sputum grew no pathogens; including on Löwenstein–Jensen medium.

1. What is the most likely diagnosis?
    a) Atypical mycobacterial infection
    b) Bronchiolitis obliterans with organizing pneumonia
    c) Alveolar cell carcinoma
    d) Inadequately treated pneumonia
    e) Cryptococcal pneumonia
    f) Large-cell carcinoma

Case 12.2

A 27-year-old Korean chef presented with a four-week history of rigors, which had persisted despite a herbal remedy. Six months before he had been prescribed chloramphenicol for conjunctivitis, which he thought was due to dirty contact lenses. On examination he was febrile and jaundiced, with a palpable liver edge. No other abnormality was detected. Blood cultures grew *Escherichia coli* in both of two sets.

1. Select the single most likely diagnosis from each of the two groups below:

    a) Ascending cholangitis
    b) Cholecystitis
    c) Pancreatitis
    d) Hepatic abscess
    e) Subphrenic abscess
    f) Hepatitis

    g) Sclerosing cholangitis
    h) *Entamoeba histolytica* infection
    i) Chloramphenicol toxicity
    j) Heavy metal poisoning
    k) *Clonorchis sinensis* infection
    l) *Acanthamoeba* infection
    m) *Paragonimus westermani* infection

Case 12.3

A 20-year-old shop assistant presented to casualty with a painful right hip. The hip had been painful for several weeks, although there was no history of trauma. She had no past medical history and took no drugs, although she said she had also suffered pain from her other hip in the past. On examination she was of African origin and her right hip was painful to move. There was also reduced range of movement in the left hip. Examination was otherwise normal.

The radiograph of the right hip is shown in the figure at the top of page 99.

Hb 9.8 g/dl, MCV 69 fl, MCH 24 pg, red cell count 8.4×10^{12}/l (normal: 3.9–5.6×10^{12}/l), white cell count 12.4×10^9/l, platelets 402×10^9/l, electrolytes normal.

1. What is the most likely underlying diagnosis?
    a) Haemoglobin C thalassaemia
    b) Haemoglobin CC disease
    c) Heterozygous sickle cell anaemia
    d) Homozygous sickle cell anaemia

e) Haemoglobin E thalassaemia
f) Sickle beta-thalassaemia

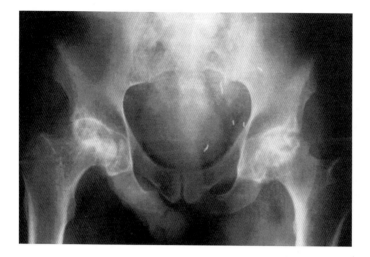

2. Which of the following findings on haemoglobin electrophoresis is most likely?
   a) 100% HbS
   b) 100% HbA
   c) 100% HbC
   d) 60% HbS, 40% HbA
   e) 40% HbS, 60% HbA
   f) 50% HbC, 50% HbA
   g) 25% HbF

Case 12.4

A 25-year-old nurse presented with an acute right hemiplegia. She had been becoming increasingly lethargic over the previous few days. While waiting to be reviewed she had a brief generalized tonic–clonic seizure, which terminated spontaneously. She had no past medical history and took no medications. On examination she was drowsy and looked ill. She was pale and had a widespread petechial rash. Her pulse was 100/min and blood pressure was 200/130 mmHg. Heart sounds were normal. Fundoscopy was normal and pupils were equal and reactive to light. There was a right homonymous hemianopia and right-sided pyramidal weakness, particularly affecting the upper limbs. Reflexes were brisk, more so on the right, with bilateral up-going plantars.

Hb 8.2 g/dl (reticulocytes 6%), white cell count 15.3 × 10⁹/l, platelets 30 × 10⁹/l, Na 128 mmol/l, K 4.8 mmol/l, urea 14.3 mmol/l, creatinine 200 μmol/l, PT 9 s (normal: 10–12 s), APTT 30 s (normal: 32–36 s), pregnancy test negative, direct Coombs' test negative.

1. Which one of the following diagnoses explains the above scenario most completely?
   a) Meningococcal septicaemia with disseminated intravascular coagulation
   b) Meningococcal septicaemia with Waterhouse–Friderichson syndrome
   c) Meningococcal meningitis complicated by cerebral infarction
   d) Haemolytic uraemic syndrome (HUS)
   e) Thrombotic thrombocytopoenic purpura (TTP)
   f) Renal artery fibromuscular dysplasia

2. Choose two treatments from the following that you would give:
   a) Anti-hypertensive agents
   b) Dexamethasone
   c) Intravenous mannitol
   d) Platelet transfusion
   e) Intravenous cefotaxime
   f) Pulsed intravenous methylprednisolone
   g) Haemodialysis
   h) Plasma exchange
   i) Intravenous hydrocortisone

Case 12.5

A 16-year-old girl presented to casualty with a painful swollen knee following a minor knock. Her past medical history was unremarkable, although on direct questioning she said that she had always bruised very easily. There was no family history. On examination she was 130 cm tall, although still prepubertal. She was not haemodynamically compromised. Her right knee was warm and swollen, with movement painful in all directions. Blood was aspirated from the joint.

Hb 13.2 g/dl, platelets 280 × 10⁹/l, PT 14 s (control 10–12 s), APTT 45 s (control 24–28 s), TT 11 s (control 9–11 s). Von Willebrand factor: within normal limits. Platelet aggregation studies normal.

1. Choose the two most likely haematological diagnoses from the following list:
   a) Haemophilia A or B
   b) Lupus anticoagulant
   c) Factor XII deficiency
   d) Prekallikrein/kininogen deficiency
   e) Factor XI deficiency
   f) Von Willebrand's disease
   g) Bernard–Soulier disease

2. Which two of the following would be included in your initial investigation?
   a) Assay clotting factors
   b) Dilute Russell's viper venom time
   c) Studies of von Willebrand factor function
   d) Serial dilution of plasma with repeat APTT/PTT
   e) Sequence fibrinogen genes
   f) Brain MRI
   g) Abdominal ultrasonography
   h) Karyotype analysis
   i) Pituitary function testing

Case 12.6

A 60-year-old man presented with abdominal pain, nausea and vomiting. He was continuing to pass flatus. Over the previous few months he had suffered with intermittent colicky abdominal pain and diarrhoea. He described occasional tenesmus. He had never noticed any blood, pallor or foul smell to his stools. In his past medical history he had a cholecystectomy eight years previously and had gradually worsening COAD. He smoked 20 cigarettes per day and drank 20–30 units of alcohol per week. On examination he was apyrexial. He was breathing with an increased respiratory rate through pursed lips. His chest was hyperexpanded, with increased resonance and poor air entry. His abdomen was distended, slightly tender in the left iliac fossa and tympanitic. There was no peritonism. Loud bowel sounds were audible. There were no hernias, and rectal examination was normal.

Full blood count, electrolytes, liver function tests and clotting were all normal. Erect CXR: emphysematous lung fields, with a rim of subdiaphragmatic free air. pO_2 10.2 kPa, pCO_2 4.4 kPa. Rigid sigmoidoscopy showed a few bluish sessile polyps in the proximal rectum with normal overlying mucosa.

His DCBE is shown in the figure at the top of page 102.

1. What is the diagnosis?
   a) Diverticulosis
   b) Diffusely infiltrating colonic tumour
   c) Ischaemic colitis
   d) Colonic pseudo-obstruction
   e) Idiopathic pneumatosis cystoides coli
   f) Peptic ulcer
   g) Ulcerative colitis

2. What would your initial treatment be?
   a) High-concentration oxygen with careful blood gas monitoring
   b) Surgical referral for emergency laparotomy
   c) Intravenous metronidazole with a third-generation cephalosporin
   d) Hyperbaric oxygen
   e) Intravenous corticosteroids

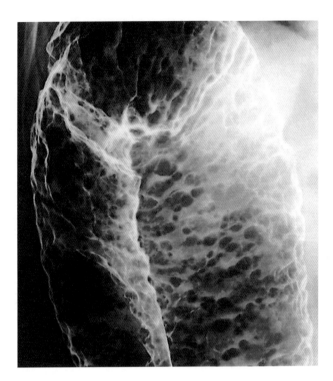

Case 12.7

A 65-year-old man had received five days of intravenous antibiotics for a *Streptococcus viridans* infection of a congenitally bicuspid aortic valve when he developed increasing breathlessness over 24 hours. At a recent insurance medical, an aortic ejection systolic murmur with normal pulse character had been noted. On examination his blood pressure was 160/60 mmHg and his pulse rate was 110/min; it was collapsing in character. His JVP was elevated to his ears, with a normal waveform. His apex beat was of normal character and undisplaced. A continuous murmur was audible at the left sternal edge, radiating widely and associated with a thrill. His chest was clear. ECG was normal. Serial CKs were normal.

1. Which two of the following diagnoses best fit the above situation?
    a) Acute mitral regurgitation
    b) Acute aortic regurgitation
    c) Ruptured sinus of Valsalva aneurysm
    d) Acute ventricular septal defect
    e) Patent ductus arteriosus
    f) Acute atrial septal defect
    g) Coronary arteriovenous shunt

Case 12.8

A 32-year-old vet was admitted with fever and shortness of breath. Hitherto well, he had returned three days before from his first trip to Malawi, where he had been undertaking a short field research project concerning cattle farming practices. During the return flight he had started to feel generally unwell, with malaise and myalgias in association with chest discomfort and a dry cough. At home he had found his temperature to be 38 °C. These symptoms had persisted for three days, during which time he had stayed off work and taken paracetamol. After feeling slightly better the previous day, he had then started to feel very unwell overnight, with rapidly progressive shortness of breath and profuse sweating.

On examination he appeared very unwell, tachypnoeic and cyanosed, with a temperature of 39 °C. There was audible inspiratory stridor and expiratory wheeze, but the chest was otherwise clear. The pulse rate was 115/min, blood pressure was 90/55 mmHg, there were no audible murmurs, and the abdomen was soft. There was mild nuchal rigidity.

PaO_2 7.6 kPa, $PaCO_2$ 3.2 kPa, pH 7.15. Hb 12.2 g/dl, white cell count 16.7 × 10^9/l (90% neutrophils), platelets 180 × 10^9/l, CRP 290 mg/l, Na 136 mM, K 4.5 mM, Cr 140 mM.

The chest radiograph showed marked, symmetrical mediastinal widening, but the lung fields were largely clear.

1. Which of the following diagnoses is most likely?
   a) Tularaemia
   b) *Mycoplasma pneumoniae* pneumonia
   c) Legionnaires' disease
   d) *Pneumocystis carinii* pneumonia
   e) Anthrax
   f) Hantavirus pneumonitis
   g) Psittacosis
   h) Q fever
   i) Miliary TB

Case 12.9

A 17-year-old man is referred on account of delayed puberty. His past history was unremarkable apart from bilateral cryptorchidism corrected surgically as a baby. He exercised only occasionally and ate well. On examination he was clinically prepubertal, with testicular volumes of 1 ml bilaterally. His weight was 60 kg. His sense of smell was impaired. Examination was otherwise normal.

There were normal cortisol and growth hormone responses to insulin-induced hypoglycaemia. Full blood count, electrolytes, liver function tests, T_4, TSH and prolactin were all normal. LH 0.3 U/l (normal: 6–13 U/l), FSH 0.2 U/l. CXR: normal. CT pituitary and hypothalamus: normal.

1. What is the most likely diagnosis?
   a) Primary testicular failure due to previous surgery
   b) Kallman's syndrome
   c) Bardet–Biedl syndrome
   d) Anorexia nervosa
   e) Sarcoidosis
   f) Klinefelter's syndrome
   g) Langerhans cell histiocytosis

2. What do you expect the karyotype to be?
   a) 46, XX
   b) 47, XXY
   c) 47, XYY
   d) 46, XY
   e) 45, X
   f) 45, X/46, XY mosaic
   g) 46, Xq-Y

Case 12.10

A 16-year-old boy presented with progressive drooping of his eyelids. There appeared to be no diurnal variation. He was otherwise well, in particular with no dysphagia. He had no past medical or family history of note. On examination he had a bilateral partial ptosis, which was not fatiguable. Pupils were round, equal-sized and normally reactive to light. There was no proptosis or chemosis. Both lateral and vertical eye movement amplitude was decreased. Full blood count, electrolytes, calcium, phosphate and CXR were all normal. ECG: 2 : 1 AV block.

1. Which of the following is the most likely diagnosis?
   a) Pituitary tumour
   b) Myasthenia gravis
   c) Myotonic dystrophy
   d) Kearns–Sayre syndrome

2. Choose one investigation from the following that you would carry out:
   a) Mitochondrial DNA analysis of blood
   b) Muscle biopsy
   c) Anti-acetylcholine receptor antibody titre
   d) Testing for CGG expansion in myotonic dystrophy gene
   e) MRI of pituitary

Exam 13

Case 13.1

A 62-year-old shopkeeper had been more breathless than usual when walking her dog since an attack of flu the previous autumn. She decided to seek medical attention when she noticed herself to be breathless climbing stairs. She was also beginning to lose weight. On direct questioning, she said she had suffered from arthritis for several years and had had an asymptomatic ventricular septal defect (VSD) since childhood. Her only medication was paracetamol and antibiotic prophylaxis when visiting the dentist. She had smoked 20 cigarettes per day for 40 years. On examination she was apyrexial with no lymphadenopathy but was clubbed. There were Bouchard's and Heberden's nodes bilaterally, but otherwise general examination was normal. The JVP was not raised and heart sounds were normal, but bibasal crepitations were audible on inspiration.

Open lung biopsy showed patchy interstitial fibrosis at varying stages, on a background of chronic inflammation. Full blood count, urea and electrolytes, and liver function indices were all normal.

CRP 30 mg/l, ESR 55 mm/h, rheumatoid factor 1/16, ANA weakly positive.

1. What is the likely diagnosis?
   a) Rheumatoid arthritis with pulmonary involvement
   b) Cryptogenic fibrosing alveolitis (CFA)
   c) Extrinsic allergic alveolitis
   d) SLE
   e) Drug-induced fibrosing alveolitis
   f) Systemic sclerosis

2. Choose one or more of the following features on plain chest radiograph that would be at odds with your diagnosis:
   a) Normal appearance of lungs
   b) Bilateral upper-zone reticulonodular shadowing
   c) Bilateral lower-zone reticulonodular shadowing
   d) Bilateral hilar lymphadenopathy
   e) Right-sided pleural effusion
   f) Extensive air bronchogram

3. What median survival for this condition would you have in mind when advising the patient further?
   a) One year
   b) Three years
   c) Six years
   d) Ten years
   e) Twenty years

Case 13.2

A 17-year-old Kosovan asylum-seeker, recently arrived in the country, was referred from the local detention centre with a sudden onset of shortness of breath and palpitation. For the past week he had been suffering a sore throat and feeling generally unwell. The GP has seen him early in the illness and noted cervical lymphadenopathy and a tonsillar membrane, and so had diagnosed glandular fever and given only paracetamol. Over the preceding 48 hours he had been feeling better. Apart from normal childhood illnesses he had otherwise been well. On examination he looked ill, with a rapid thready pulse, raised JVP, low blood pressure and displaced volume-loaded apex beat. He had a gallop rhythm, with clinical mitral regurgitation and tricuspid regurgitation on auscultation. His liver was palpable. The 12-lead ECG showed inferolateral T-wave inversion, with prolonged PR and QT intervals.

1. What is the most likely diagnosis?
   a) EBV-induced myocarditis
   b) Acute retroviral syndrome
   c) Adenovirus-induced myocarditis
   d) Group A *Streptococcal* pharyngitis and rheumatic fever
   e) Diphtheritic myocarditis
   f) Kawasaki disease

Case 13.3

A 35-year-old lady presented with an axillary vein thrombosis. She was waiting to see a gastroenterologist on account of increasing fatigue and intermittent abdominal pain over the last three years. She had no previous medical history or family history and had never taken any medications, except for paracetamol for occasional headaches. On examination she was mildly jaundiced but examination was otherwise normal.

Hb 9.8 g/dl, white cell count 1.8×10^9/l (neutrophils 40%, lymphocytes 60%), platelets 130×10^9/l, ESR 24 mm/h. ANA, rheumatoid factor, anti-dsDNA and antiphospholipid antibodies: all negative. Urine dipstick positive for blood.

1. What is the most likely diagnosis?
   a) Paroxysmal nocturnal haemoglobinuria (PNH)
   b) Beçhet's disease
   c) Lymphoproliferative disorder with haemolytic anaemia
   d) Paraneoplastic hypercoagulability
   e) SLE
   f) Factor V Leiden

2. Which of the following tests is most likely to yield the definitive diagnosis?
   a) Iron studies
   b) Direct Coombs' test
   c) Bone marrow aspiration and trephine
   d) Serum haptoglobins
   e) Urine microscopy
   f) MRI of abdomen
   g) Addition of acidified serum to red cells

Case 13.4

A 16-year-old woman presented with an insidious onset of hearing difficulties, incoordination, and hand and feet paraesthesiae. Her symptoms became dramatically worse when she started to diet. Her past medical history was unremarkable, although she had developed dry and scaling skin over the previous year.

1. What is the likely diagnosis?
   a) Mixed thiamine and riboflavin deficiency
   b) Spinocerebellar degeneration
   c) Refsum's disease
   d) Multiple sclerosis

2. Choose one investigation from the following that you would carry out:
   a) Thiamine levels
   b) MRI brain
   c) Lumbar puncture, including oligoclonal bands
   d) Plasma phytanic acid levels

Case 13.5

A 20-year-old man presented with shortness of breath and an increase in his sputum production. He was feverish. He suffered chest infections three or four times per year, and even when well he produced copious amounts of green sputum. He had been rendered wheelchair-bound at the age of 10, a slowly progressive clumsiness and instability having started in early childhood. He was adopted but had managed to discover that an uncle and a great-uncle had died young and wheelchair-bound.

His CXR is shown here:

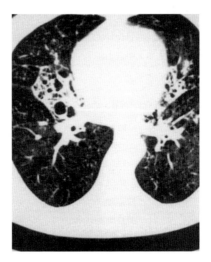

1. Why is he wheelchair-bound?
   a) Bronchiectasis
   b) Ataxia telangiectasia
   c) Hereditary spinocerebellar degeneration
   d) Cystic fibrosis

Case 13.6

A 72-year-old man was referred by his GP with abnormal liver function tests and abdominal swelling. In clinic, his complaints were of three months of anorexia, fatigue and abdominal swelling, as well as increasing shortness of breath on exertion. He had been short of breath for many years on account of his 20 per day smoking habit. He drank alcohol only occasionally. His past history was notable only for a two-vessel coronary artery bypass graft (CABG) some nine years before, since when he had been angina-free. He had never suffered an MI. On examination his pulse was 80/min, regular and of normal character, and his blood pressure was 140/80 mmHg. His heart sounds were quiet but a third heart sound was heard. His JVP was raised above the angle of his jaw. His chest was hyperexpanded, with occasional inspiratory crepitations clearing on coughing. He had 5-cm smooth hepatomegaly and moderate ascites, but no stigmata of chronic liver disease and no splenomegaly. He had mildly swollen ankles.

Full blood count and electrolytes were normal. Albumin 28 g/l, bilirubin 30 μmol/l, ALT 80 U/l, ALP 290 U/l. Hepatitis B surface antigen was negative. Posteroanterior CXR was reported as being unremarkable. Conventional 12-lead and right-sided lead ECGs: non-specific T-wave inversion only.

1. Select the most likely diagnosis from the following:
   a) Budd–Chiari syndrome
   b) Cryptogenic liver cirrhosis
   c) Chronic autoimmune hepatitis
   d) Transfusion-acquired hepatitis C infection
   e) Restrictive cardiomyopathy
   f) Constrictive pericarditis

2. Select the single definitive investigation from the following:
   a) Percutaneous liver biopsy
   b) Liver autoantibodies and immunoglobulin levels
   c) Transthoracic echocardiography
   d) Transoesophageal echocardiography
   e) Cardiac catheterization
   f) Hepatitis C PCR
   g) Abdominal ultrasonography with Doppler traces

Case 13.7

A 32-year-old lady developed sudden-onset left flank pain while on a desert camel trek. After the pain had subsided she passed a small stone in her urine. She was otherwise well, with no past medical or family history. She took no drugs. On return to the UK she was investigated. General examination was normal.

Electrolytes were normal. Corrected calcium 2.4 mmol/l, phosphate 1.1 mmol/l, albumin 42 g/l, ALP 100 U/l, ALT 16 U/l, magnesium 1.0 mmol/l, PTH 4.8 pmol/l (normal: 0.9–5.4 pmol/l). Blood pH 7.37. TSH, CXR, abdominal X-ray and IVP were all normal. Urinalysis: normal. 24-hour urinary calcium: 12 mmol/day (normal: 2.5–7.5 mmol/day). No amino aciduria.

1. What is the diagnosis?
   a) Medullary sponge kidney
   b) Idiopathic hypercalciuria
   c) Sarcoidosis
   d) Distal renal tubular acidosis
   e) Medullary sponge kidney

2. Which one or more of the following treatments should be recommended?
   a) Increase fluid intake to 5–6 l/day
   b) Decrease sodium and protein in diet

c) Increase sodium and potassium in the diet
d) Long-acting thiazide diuretic
e) Triamterene
f) Regular loop diuretic
g) Spironolactone

Case 13.8

A 20-year-old student presented with a three-day history of increasing malaise and headache. She felt sick and had a painful neck. She was febrile. An urgent CT followed by a lumbar puncture were carried out. Both were normal, but on account of a raised ESR she was followed up in clinic. In clinic she complained of non-specific tiredness and some shortness of breath on exercise. However, her repeat ESR was normal so she was discharged from clinic. Her lassitude persisted over the next year, and she was eventually referred back with the additional symptom of pain in her legs on running. She was found to be hypertensive, with a blood pressure of 180/110 mmHg. Femoral pulses were weak, with a radiofemoral delay. An abdominal bruit was heard.

1. What is the most likely diagnosis?
   a) Superinfection of congenital aortic coarctation
   b) Giant cell arteritis
   c) Kawasaki disease
   d) Takayasu's arteritis
   e) Moya moya disease
   f) Buerger's disease
   g) Fibromuscular dysplasia
   h) Retroperitoneal fibrosis

2. Select the most appropriate investigation from the following:
   a) Temporal artery biopsy
   b) Renal biopsy
   c) Aortography
   d) Abdominal ultrasonography
   e) Cerebral angiography
   f) Serial blood cultures

Case 13.9

A 20-year-old nurse presented with a two-year history of excessive thirst, polyuria and nocturia. Her weight had increased by nearly 20 kg in that period. Her development had been normal and she maintained regular menses. Indeed, she was otherwise fit and well. Past medical, family and drug histories were unremarkable. Full examination was entirely normal. Full blood count, electrolytes, glucose, calcium, phosphate, ALT, ALP and CXR were all normal.

Results of water deprivation test were as follows:

Time	Weight (kg)	Plasma osmolality (mosmol/kg)	Urine volume (ml)	Urine osmolality (mosmol/kg)
08.30	90.3	296	–	–
11.30	88.8	300	320	92
13.30	87.8	308	230	114

1. What is the most accurate diagnosis based on these results?
   a) Dipsogenic diabetes insipidus
   b) Nephrogenic diabetes insipidus
   c) Hypothalamic diabetes insipidus
   d) Diabetes insipidus
   e) Interstitial renal disease

2. Which investigation would come next?
   a) Hypertonic saline infusion with serial ADH determination
   b) Urine calcium determination
   c) Urine osmolality after desmopressin
   d) Short synacthen test
   e) CT hypothalamus
   f) Ellsworth–Howard test

Case 13.10

A 36-year-old lady presented with double vision. Several weeks before she had developed a droopy face, which her GP had diagnosed as Bell's palsy. She had also had several episodes of painful, swollen knees and on one occasion a painful wrist. Now, in addition to her double vision, she had a headache and felt nauseated. Prior to these symptoms she had been well, with no past medical or family history of note. On examination she had mild meningism and a partial right third nerve palsy. The facial palsy appeared to have resolved. Both knee joints were painful and swollen. Examination was otherwise normal.

Her ECG is shown in the following figure:

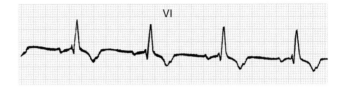

Full blood count, electrolytes, liver function tests and CXR were all normal. CT head was normal.

CSF: protein 1.2 g/l, 105×10^6 white cells (98% lymphocytes), no organisms.

1. What is the most likely diagnosis?
   a) Sarcoidosis
   b) Behçet's syndrome
   c) Lyme disease
   d) Whipple's disease
   e) SLE
   f) Reiter's syndrome

Exam 14

Case 14.1

A 53-year-old insurance salesman was referred to clinic with breathlessness. He had begun to wheeze following a general anaesthetic for a submucosal resection four months previously. A troublesome cough prompted his GP to prescribe a course of oral prednisolone, with good effect. However, his symptoms recurred on stopping the prednisolone, with poorer control being obtained with inhaled beclomethasone and salbutamol. In clinic he commented that he had been feeling less well recently, with intermittent fevers and some weight loss. He had made no foreign trips recently and had no relevant past medical history. He was homosexual. There was no history of personal or family atopy. His temperature was 37.7 °C but examination was otherwise normal.

Hb 14.5 g/dl, white cell count 9.8 × 10^9/l (53% neutrophils, 31% lymphocytes), ESR 110 mm/h, urea 5.4 mmol/l, creatinine 98 μmol/l. Skin test battery to inhaled allergens, including *Aspergillus fumigatus*: negative. Urine dipstick normal. Serum IgE normal. Serological screen for parasitic infection negative. Static and dynamic pulmonary function tests within normal limits.

His chest radiograph is shown here:

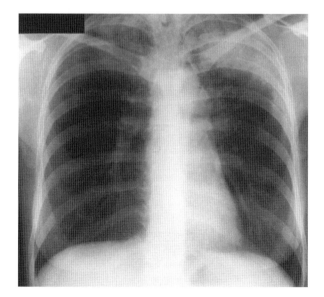

1. What is the most likely diagnosis?
    a) *Pneumocystis carinii* pneumonia
    b) Churg–Strauss syndrome
    c) Cryptococcal pneumonia
    d) Chronic eosinophilic pneumonia
    e) Wegener's granulomatosis

2. What is the treatment?
    a) Nebulized pentamidine
    b) Oral corticosteroids
    c) Highly active anti-retroviral therapy (HAART)
    d) Intravenous amphotericin B
    e) Co-trimoxazole

Case 14.2

A 41-year-old lawyer presented with a 10-week history of increasingly severe, foul-smelling diarrhoea. She reported no blood or mucus and only minimal abdominal discomfort and swelling. She had felt nauseated but had not vomited. Her energy levels and appetite were decreased. She lived in London during the week and spent the weekends at her French residence. There was no other history of foreign travel. Her past medical history was unremarkable. On examination she was thin. Apart from an erythematous anal mucosa, no abnormality was detected.

Sigmoidoscopy and rectal biopsy did not suggest intrinsic colonic disease, and OGD with duodenal biopsy was normal.

Na 130 mmol/l, K 2.6 mmol/l, urea 12.6 mmol/l, creatinine 110 μmol/l, total calcium 2.4 mmol/l, phosphate 0.8 mmol/l, albumin 30 g/l, ALT 28 U/l. HIV test: negative. Full blood count, clotting and CXR: all normal. Stool Na 90 mmol/l, K 40 mmol/l, osmolality 260 mosmol/kg (normal: <350 mosmol/kg). Lactose hydrogen breath test normal.

Consider the following possible diagnoses and investigations:

a) Laxative abuse
b) Verner–Morrison syndrome
c) Zollinger–Ellison syndrome
d) Glucagonoma
e) Medullary carcinoma of thyroid
f) Giardiasis
g) Small-bowel carcinoma
h) Chronic salmonellosis

A) Urine laxative screen
B) Stool laxative screen
C) Fasting gut hormones

D) Pentagastrin stimulation test
E) Stool immunoassay
F) Secretin stimulation test
G) Blood cultures
H) Abdominal ultrasound examination

For each alternative piece of information below, select the single most likely diagnosis and the single investigation most likely to be diagnostic (each option may be selected once, more than once, or not at all):

1. The colonic mucosa on sigmoidoscopy appeared diffusely pigmented.
2. The patient had a family history of MEN1.
3. The patient later admitted that she had been suffering a pruritic rash on the backs of her shoulders, appearing as lichenoid plaques and papules on examination.
4. The patient is found to carry a germ-line mutation in the *ret* proto-oncogene.
5. The patient later recalls that a number of friends had had a similar, but acute and self-limiting, illness at the start of her own symptoms.

Case 14.3

A 76-year-old man presented with near-total blindness coming on over half an hour. On examination his visual acuity was correctable to 6/6 in each eye, but only the very central area of vision was present. Fundi were normal and pupils were equal and normally reactive to light.

1. Select the most likely diagnosis from the following:
    a) Retinitis pigmentosa
    b) Pituitary apoplexy
    c) Midbrain infarct
    d) Bilateral posterior cerebral artery infarct
    e) Hysteria

Case 14.4

A 48-year-old lady was referred to the out-patients department with a two-year history of refractory hypertension. She was currently taking atenolol and slow-release nifedipine. She had no past medical history. Examination was normal. Full blood count, ESR, electrolytes, CXR, ECG, MSU and IVP were all normal. She was commenced on an ACE inhibitor, but this had to be stopped on account of a troublesome cough. Control was eventually gained with a combination of atenolol and hydralazine. One month later she presented with a rash, pleuritic chest pain and fevers. On examination she had a widespread erythematous rash and was febrile. A left-sided pleural rub was audible. Examination was otherwise normal.

1. What is the most likely diagnosis?
   a) Idiopathic SLE
   b) Still's disease
   c) Microscopic polyangiitis
   d) Hydralazine-induced lupus
   e) Atenolol-induced lupus

2. Choose one of the following investigations to support this diagnosis:
   a) Punch biopsy of skin
   b) ANCA
   c) Anti-dsDNA antibody
   d) Anti-ribonucleoprotein (RNP) antibody
   e) Anti-histone antibody
   f) Anti-centromere antibody
   g) Anti-Jo

Case 14.5

A 30-year-old hairdresser gave birth to a healthy, normal-looking baby boy after an uneventful pregnancy and labour. During the first day of life he was noticed to become irritable, and on the second day he began having difficult-to-control seizures. Pyridoxine 100 mg had no effect. Postictal examination was normal. He remained afebrile. Full blood count, electrolytes, calcium, phosphate, magnesium, glucose, arterial blood gases, serum ammonia, urine and blood amino acids, organic acids, CT head and CSF analysis were all normal. There was no serological evidence of any infection with toxoplasmosis, herpes, rubella, CMV, syphilis or Coxsackie virus. His mother was not unduly concerned; when confronted, she said that the same thing had happened to her other two children but that they had both settled down soon and were now fit and well.

1. Select the two most likely diagnoses from the following list:
   a) Withdrawal fits
   b) Benign familial convulsions
   c) Munchausen's-by-proxy
   d) Pyridoxine-sensitive seizures
   e) Phenylketonuria

Case 14.6

A 28-year-old labourer presented with a four-day history of severe muscle aches, worst in his calves and back. He also complained of a severe frontal headache, nausea, and hot and cold spells. His past medical history was unremarkable, and he had not left the UK for some years. On examination he looked ill and mildly jaundiced.

His temperature was 38 °C. He had pronounced conjunctival suffusion and a faint maculopapular rash. A liver edge was palpable. His pulse rate was 100/min and blood pressure was 110/60 mmHg. An ejection systolic murmur was audible at the lower left sternal edge. Examination was otherwise normal.

Clotting studies were normal. Urea 10.2 mmol/l, creatinine 190 μmol/l, albumin 29 g/l, bilirubin 35 μM, ALT 140 U/l, ALP 220 U/l. Urinalysis: protein +, blood +, ketones ++. CXR: patchy bibasal alveolar shadowing. ECG: normal.

1. What is the most likely diagnosis?
    a) Hepatitis A infection
    b) Hepatitis B infection
    c) Hantavirus infection
    d) Leptospirosis
    e) Lyme disease
    f) Tick-borne relapsing fever

2. Which of the following is true?
    a) Blood and urine cultures in week one should grow the causative organism
    b) Urine cultures in week two should grow the causative organism
    c) Blood cultures in week two should grow the causative organism
    d) There is a >50% chance of hepatic encephalopathy developing
    e) There is a >50% chance of a Jarisch–Herxheimer reaction following treatment
    f) Beta-lactam antibiotics will be ineffective

Case 14.7

A 75-year-old lady presented with presyncope after the passage of several melaena stools. She had no preceding gastrointestinal symptoms. For the previous 18 years she had suffered intermittent joint aches affecting her wrists, ankles and fingers. On examination she looked pale. Her arm is shown below:

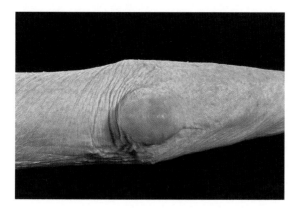

Her pulse was 110/min and regular. Blood pressure was 120/80 mmHg, dropping to 90/60 mmHg on standing. Heart sounds were normal. A 5-cm spleen was palpable, but there was no other organomegaly.

Hb 8.4 g/dl, platelets 150×10^9/l, INR 1.2. Electrolytes: normal.

1. Which two of the following suggest that the joint symptoms and splenomegaly are linked?
   a) Neutropenia
   b) Reed–Sternberg cells on splenic biopsy
   c) A history of NSAID use
   d) HLA-B27 positivity
   e) 3.4 g of proteinuria in 24 hours
   f) Dry bone marrow aspirates
   g) Scaling maculopapular lesions in the natal cleft and on the knees

Case 14.8

A 36-year-old lady presented with a repetitive nodding movement of her head and increasing weakness and stiffness of her legs. Five years ago she recalled a period of about a week when her legs were weak but got better before she managed to get an appointment to see her GP. Two years after that she developed double vision for three weeks. This recurred four years after this, in addition with a misting of the vision of the left eye. She had no other symptoms. She had never had any mouth or genital ulcers, respiratory or gastrointestinal symptoms, venereal disease or tick bites. There were no autoimmune symptoms. Past medical and family history was unremarkable. She took no medications. General examination was normal. Higher mental function was normal. Visual acuity was 6/12 in the left eye and 6/18 in the right. She could see only seven Ishihara charts with the left eye and four with the right. There was a right afferent pupillary defect. Both discs were pale. A left internuclear ophthalmoplegia (INO) was evident. She was titubating and had cerebellar speech. There were no other brainstem signs. Upper limb examination was normal except for some past pointing and dysdiadochokinesis, equal on both sides. A grade 3/5 spastic paraparesis was evident in the lower limbs, with brisk reflexes and up-going plantars. Sensation was impaired to L1. Full blood count, electrolytes, liver function tests, Igs, serum ACE and CXR were all normal. ANA, anti-dsDNA and rheumatoid factor were all negative.

At two-month follow-up her lower limb signs were much improved, although she continued to have cerebellar signs and titubation. Over the next 10 years she had three further episodes of double vision and leg weakness, before re-presenting with arm paraesthesiae and weakness. On examination she still had impaired colour vision and visual acuity but no INO. She continued to titubate and had upper- and lower-limb cerebellar signs. There was wasting of her right biceps, with corresponding weakness, a decreased biceps jerk and increased triceps jerk. Left elbow extension was weak, with a diminished triceps jerk. Patchy numbness could be detected over the fingers to pinprick and light touch. Spastic, weak legs were once again in evidence.

1. With regards to her most recent presentation, select the two most likely diagnoses from the following:
   a) Sarcoidosis
   b) Multiple sclerosis
   c) Cervical myelopathy
   d) Lyme disease
   e) Syphilis
   f) Arteriovenous malformation (AVM)
   g) Behçet's disease

2. Select the most pertinent investigation from the following:
   a) Nerve conduction studies
   b) Visual evoked responses
   c) MRI cervical cord
   d) MRI head

Case 14.9

A 19-year-old student was referred with increasing lethargy. Over the last nine months she had progressively lost weight despite a good appetite. She had a tendency to constipation and sometimes felt bloated after meals. She had no abdominal pain and gave no history of steatorrhoea. There was never any blood or mucus with her stools. Six months previously her periods had stopped, having previously been regular. Her childhood development had been normal, with no past medical or family history. She took no drugs and had no risk factors for HIV carriage. On examination she was very thin but of adult stature (5' 8"). Genitalia and breasts were normal. Axillary and pubic hair was present. Her skin was slightly dry and her hands and feet cool. There was minimal ankle oedema. Pulse was 60/min and blood pressure was 100/60 mmHg. JVP was not raised and heart sounds were normal. The appearance of her back is shown here:

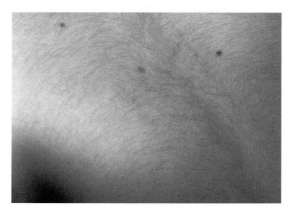

Hb 11.7 g/dl, white cell count 3.5×10^9/l, platelets 180×10^9/l, MCV 88 fl, albumin 36 g/l, ALT 20 mmol/l. Serum B12, red cell folate and iron studies all normal. TSH 1.5 mU/l, free T_3 1.8 pmol/l (normal: 3.3–8.2 pmol/l), PRL 220 mU/l, plasma 17-β-oestradiol 40 pmol/l (normal: 75–260 pmol/l), LH <0.8 U/l, FSH <0.8 U/l, cholesterol 6.5 mmol/l. 9 a.m. plasma cortisol 480 nmol/l with normal response to 250 μg synacthen. 9 a.m. GH 28 mU/l (normal: <20 mU/l).

1. What is the most likely unifying diagnosis?
   a) Polyglandular autoimmune syndrome
   b) Anorexia nervosa
   c) Hypogonadotrophic hypogonadism
   d) Primary hypothyroidism
   e) Growth-hormone-secreting pituitary adenoma
   f) Non-functioning pituitary adenoma
   g) Premature ovarian failure

Case 14.10

A 14-year-old boy presented with pain and blindness in his right eye. Over the previous few days he had felt unwell, with malaise, fevers and myalgia. He had no cough, shortness of breath, diarrhoea, abdominal discomfort, urinary frequency or dysuria. On examination he was febrile at 38.4 °C. Inflamed needle-track marks were seen in his antecubital fossae. There were no stigmata of infective endocarditis. Heart sounds were normal and his chest was clear. There was no organomegaly. Visual acuity was 6/5 in the left eye but only light perception remained in the left. There was a left afferent pupillary defect.

This was his eye:

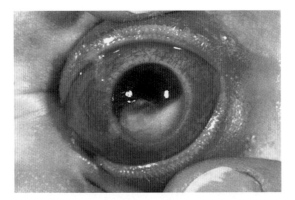

CXR, ECG, and transthoracic and transoesophageal echocardiograms were all normal.

1. What is the most likely diagnosis?
   a) Retinal vasculitis
   b) Posterior uveitis
   c) Metastatic bacterial endophthalmitis
   d) Metastatic bacterial panophthalmitis
   e) Fungal endophthalmitis

Exam 15

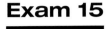

Case 15.1

A 65-year-old lady presented with increasing jaundice, pale stools and dark urine. She had suffered no weight loss, abdominal pain, pruritus or fevers. She felt slightly nauseated, but her appetite was good. She had had no infectious contacts, no previous blood transfusions, no episodes of jaundice, and no recent foreign travel. She smoked 10 cigarettes per day but drank alcohol only occasionally. She went through the menopause at the age of 32. On examination she was icteric but with no signs of chronic liver disease and no lymphadenopathy. She was afebrile. Her upper abdomen was slightly tender, with a mass palpable in the right upper quadrant, which descended on inspiration. Bowel sounds and rectal examination were both normal.

Hb 11.6 g/dl, white cell count 9.7 × 10⁹/l, platelets 420 × 10⁹/l, PT 12 s (normal: 10–12 s), Na 139 mmol/l, K 4.2 mmol/l, urea 5.4 mmol/l, creatinine 98 μmol/l, albumin 36 g/l, bilirubin 120 μmol/l, ALT 80 U/l, ALP 290 U/l, GGT 330 U/l. Bilirubinuria. Abdominal X-ray: no calcification, soft tissue shadow right upper quadrant.

1. Which of the following could explain the biochemistry and examination findings?
   a) Liver fluke infestation
   b) Primary sclerosing cholangitis
   c) Primary biliary cirrhosis
   d) Carcinoma of pancreas
   e) Carcinoma of bile duct
   f) Common bile duct gallstone

2. Which of the above is most likely?

Case 15.2

A 33-year-old sewage worker presented to eye casualty with a lump on his right eye, which had enlarged over a few days. On examination a granulomatous lesion was evident on the conjunctiva. Tender pre-auricular lymph nodes were palpable, and a small crusted papule on his right forearm where his new kitten had scratched him was seen. He was otherwise well, with no past medical history.

1. What is the diagnosis?
   a) Parinaud's oculoglandular syndrome
   b) Weil's disease
   c) Sarcoid

Case 15.3

A 20-year-old student presented with a 24-hour history of gradual-onset double vision and tongue pain. He felt generally unwell. He was a geography student and had returned recently from an Arctic expedition, where he had had a bout of gastroenteritis just before returning home. His past medical history was unremarkable, although he did have an aunt with thyroid disease. He took no drugs. On examination his eyelids and conjunctivae were swollen. There was no lymphadenopathy or rash. He was febrile at 38.2 °C, with a blood pressure of 120/80 mmHg and pulse of 120/min. Heart sounds were normal and JVP was not raised. His apex beat was undisplaced and of normal character. Respiratory and abdominal examinations were normal. Higher mental function was normal. Pupils were equal-sized and reactive to light and accommodation. Fundi were normal. He had a complex bilateral ophthalmoplegia, with impaired eye movements bilaterally in all directions. Facial sensation was normal and corneal reflexes intact. Facial movements were normal, as were palatal movement and sensation. He was dysarthric, with weak tongue movements bilaterally. The jaw jerk was normal, as were sternocleidomastoid and trapezius strength. The remainder of the neurological examination was normal.

Hb 13.4 g/dl, white cell count 16.6×10^9/l (55% neutrophils, 26% lymphocytes), platelets 440×10^9/l. Electrolytes, liver function, calcium and phosphate were all normal. CXR was normal.

1. What is the diagnosis?
   a) Dermatomyositis
   b) Inclusion body myositis
   c) Trichinosis
   d) Myositis
   e) Vitamin A toxicity
   f) Grave's ophthalmopathy
   g) Myasthenia gravis

2. Choose one investigation from the following that you would carry out:
   a) CT orbits
   b) X-ray orbits
   c) Muscle biopsy
   d) *Trichinella* serology
   e) CT/MRI brainstem
   f) T_4/TSH

g) Vitamin A levels
h) Tensilon test

Case 15.4

A 20-year-old lady presented with a one-year history of non-bloody diarrhoea inter-spersed with brief periods of constipation. She had no nausea or vomiting but had lost some weight. Sometimes the diarrhoea was associated with colicky left upper quadrant pain. On examination she was thin and clubbed. No other abnormality was detected.

Na 138 mmol/l, K 2.9 mmol/l, urea 4.5 mmol/l, Hb 12.7 g/dl, white cell count 5.6 × 10⁹/l. Barium follow-through: normal. OGD and small-bowel biopsy: normal. Barium enema: some loss of haustrations. Sigmoidoscopy: slightly erythematous but otherwise normal-looking mucosa.

A trial of olsalazine with prednisolone showed no benefit. During a particularly severe bout of diarrhoea, she was admitted to hospital for bowel rest with intra-venous fluids for 72 hours. The diarrhoea persisted.

1. Select the two most likely diagnoses from the following:
   a) Somatostatinoma
   b) Food allergy
   c) Crohn's disease
   d) Lactose intolerance
   e) Laxative abuse
   f) Bile acid diarrhoea
   g) VIPoma
   h) Coeliac disease
   i) Irritable bowel syndrome
   j) Acute intermittent porphyria
   k) Hyperthyroidism

Case 15.5

A 40-year-old air traffic controller was admitted for elective varicose vein stripping. She had no past medical history, apart from headaches, and no relevant family history. However, her preoperative electrolytes showed a urea of 27.5 mmol/l and creatinine of 320 mmol/l. Ultrasound showed bilateral small, scarred kidneys. Red and white cells were seen on microscopy but no organisms. Two years later she re-presented with haematuria and a brief episode of left loin pain. She thought the pain had been relieved with the passage of a small blood clot. Over the next two years she gradually approached end-stage renal failure, although she continued to pass plenty of urine. Indeed, it was not possible to lower her sodium excretion below 120 mmol/24 hours.

1. What is the most likely diagnosis?
   a) Sickle cell trait
   b) Chronic obstructive uropathy
   c) IgA nephropathy
   d) Analgesic nephropathy
   e) Chronic pyelonephritis
   f) Focal segmental glomerulosclerosis
   g) Renal tuberculosis

Case 15.6

A 46-year-old lady presented with a three-month history of lethargy, anorexia and nausea. She had an ache in her loins and lower back. She had no other symptoms apart from long-standing migraines. A full examination was normal except for a blood pressure of 160/100 mmHg.

Hb 10.2 g/dl, white cell count 8.6×10^9/l, platelets 230×10^9/l, urea 22.3 mmol/l, creatinine 290 μmol/l, ESR 65 mm/h. Urine dipstick and microscopy: normal. Ultrasound: normal-sized kidneys but evidence of bilateral pelvicalyceal dilation.

1. What is the most likely diagnosis?
   a) Renal cell carcinoma
   b) Transitional cell carcinoma
   c) Analgesic nephropathy
   d) Methysergide-induced retroperitoneal fibrosis
   e) Sumatriptan-induced retroperitoneal fibrosis
   f) Bilateral hydronephrosis
   g) Takayasu's arteritis
   h) Xanthogranulomatous pyelonephritis

Case 15.7

A 27-year-old lady was admitted to hospital with a 48-hour history of profuse non-bloody diarrhoea and vomiting. She felt presyncopal but not feverish. She had no other symptoms. There was no history of shellfish or egg intake and no contact with similarly ill people. She had no relevant past medical or family history and took no drugs (including the contraceptive pill). She was married with one child, had no pets, and had made only one foreign trip recently, to Spain six months previously. On examination she was very dehydrated, with a postural drop from 100/60 mmHg to 60/40 mmHg. Her pulse was 110/min and her JVP was not visible. There was no rash. A grade 2/6 ejection systolic murmur was audible at the lower left sternal edge. She had mild epigastric tenderness. The remainder of the examination was normal.

At sigmoidoscopy loose stools were seen but no mucosal abnormality. She was resuscitated overnight. The following morning she found talking and movement of her limbs difficult. Higher mental function was normal. Visual acuity and fields, pupillary responses and eye movements were normal. Corneal reflexes were intact and no clear sensory deficit to pinprick was discernible in either the face or peripheries. Palatal and facial movements were severely diminished. There was a flaccid quadriparesis, with absent reflexes. General examination was normal, however, with no postural drop. Over the next three days, some strength returned. Spasticity was noted, the reflexes becoming brisk and the plantars up-going.

1. What is the most likely diagnosis?
   a) Midbrain infarct
   b) Medullary infarct
   c) Pontine infarct
   d) Locked-in syndrome
   e) Multiple sclerosis
   f) Central pontine myelinolysis
   g) Acute intermittent porphyria
   h) Guillain–Barré syndrome

Case 15.8

A 28-year-old saleswoman attended for her first insurance medical. Apart from what were described by her GP as intermittent panic attacks, she had no past medical history of note. She felt well and general examination was normal. However, her blood tests were abnormal: urea 4. 4 mmol/l, creatinine 87 µmol/l, corrected calcium 1.7 mmol/l, phosphate 2.0 mmol/l, albumin 40 g/l, PTH 10.5 pmol/l (normal: <0.9–5.4 pmol/l).

1. Which one or more of the following could explain these findings?
   a) Hypomagnesaemia
   b) Hypoparathyroidism
   c) Vitamin D deficiency
   d) Pseudohypoparathyroidism
   e) Pseudopseudohypoparathyroidism
   f) Di George syndrome

2. Choose one or more tests that are necessary to confirm your diagnosis:
   a) Chromosomal fluorescent in situ hybridization
   b) 24-hour urine calcium and phosphate
   c) Urinary cAMP and phosphate response to PTH infusion
   d) Urinary cAMP response to calcium infusion

e) Parathyroid autoantibodies
f) Serum magnesium
g) Serum 25-hydroxy-vitamin D

Case 15.9

A 29-year-old woman was referred due to excessive hair growth over the last 18 months. Her development had been normal to age 17, with menarche at the age of 12. Her menses were regular and lasted four days. Her libido was normal. She took no drugs but smoked 10 cigarettes per day and drank 10 units of alcohol per week. She denied illicit drug use. There was no relevant family history. On examination she was 1.75 m in height, weighed 70 kg, and had well-developed musculature. There was some temporal recession of her hair, although she tied back her hair tightly. She was not Cushingoid and she appeared euthyroid. She had abnormal hair growth on her chin, upper lip, chest and abdomen. Her voice was deep. Vaginal examination was normal but the clitoris was enlarged. There was no postural blood pressure drop. The remainder of the examination was normal.

Full blood count, electrolytes and liver function tests were normal. Plasma testosterone 9.7 nmol/l (normal: 1–2.5 nmol/l).

1. Choose the two most likely diagnoses from the following:
    a) Cushing's syndrome
    b) Adrenal tumour
    c) Polycystic ovary syndrome (PCOS)
    d) Ovarian tumour
    e) Non-classical congenital adrenal hyperplasia (CAH)
    f) Testicular feminization
    g) Familial hirsutism
    h) Severe insulin resistance
    i) Hyperprolactinaemia

2. Which two of the following investigations would be most informative?
    a) 24-hour urinary free cortisol
    b) GnRH stimulation test
    c) Dexamethasone suppression test
    d) Midnight 17-hydroxy-progesterone
    e) Oral glucose tolerance testing with insulin measurement
    f) LH, FSH and oestradiol determination
    g) Prolactin determination
    h) Pituitary MRI
    i) Abdominal CT
    j) Transvaginal ultrasound

Case 15.10

A 50-year old man presented with back pain. Initial test results were as follows:
Na 124 mmol/l, K 3.5 mmol/l, chloride 94 mmol/l, urea 15.5 mmol/l, creatinine 200 μmol/l, bicarbonate 22 mmol/l, glucose 5.5 mmol/l, plasma osmolality 290 mosmol/kg. Urinalysis: no protein.

1. What is the most likely cause of the renal failure?
   a) Hyperparathyroidism
   b) Renal cell carcinoma
   c) Pyelonephritis
   d) Myeloma
   e) Retroperitoneal fibrosis
   f) Analgesic nephropathy
   g) Metastatic carcinoma

Exam 16

■■■■■■■■■

Case 16.1

A 26-year-old shop assistant had been suffering from intermittent pain and tenderness affecting her elbows, wrists, knees and ankles for the last two years, symptomatic relief being obtained from NSAIDs. For the last two months she had been feeling increasingly unwell, with fever, weight loss, a non-productive cough and left-sided pleuritic chest pain. She smoked 20 cigarettes per day. On examination her temperature was 37.9 °C. The synovium was easily palpable over her wrists and metacarpophalangeal joints, which were also tender. No subcutaneous nodules were detected. Her left lower zone was dull to percussion, with quiet breath sounds. The CXR was reported as showing a moderate left-sided pleural effusion in addition to reticular shadowing in the left apex.

Aspiration revealed turbid, straw-coloured fluid with a protein content of 48 g/l and glucose content of 1.4 mmol/l. It contained many lymphocytes but no malignant cells. Culture was sterile at five days.

1. What is the most likely cause of the effusion?
   a) Sarcoidosis
   b) Rheumatoid arthritis
   c) Tuberculosis
   d) Still's disease
   e) Lymphoma
   f) Lung carcinoma

2. Which one of the following investigations would be most likely to be diagnostic?
   a) High-resolution CT chest
   b) Mantoux test
   c) Pleural biopsy
   d) Rheumatoid factor
   e) Serum ACE
   f) Transbronchial lung biopsy

Case 16.2

A 44-year-old lawyer with cirrhosis due to hepatitis C infection developed rigors with abdominal pain and vomiting. He had returned that day from a business trip to the southern USA, and his last meal, some 18 hours before, had been a salad of raw oysters and prawns. On examination he looked ill. His temperature was 39.5 °C, pulse was 120/min and thready, and blood pressure was 90/50 mmHg. His apex beat was hyperdynamic but no murmurs were audible. A 12-lead ECG was normal. Blood cultures grew a motile, curved, Gram-negative bacillus. He needed ICU admission, where invasive studies showed a high cardiac output with very low systemic vascular resistance. On the day following admission, he developed erythematous patches on his legs, which progressed quickly to bullae.

1. What is the diagnosis?
    a) *Campylobacter* septicaemia
    b) Cholera
    c) Typhoid fever
    d) Toxin-mediated gastroenteritis with commensal contamination of blood culture
    e) *Vibrio parahaemolyticus* septicaemia
    f) *Vibrio vulnificus* septicaemia

Case 16.3

A 76-year-old woman presented with severe right knee pain developing over two to three weeks. She could recall no trauma. She had had no fevers, sweats or constitutional disturbance. She suffered stable angina and had undergone hysterectomy for uterine bleeding in her fifties. She was also awaiting a hepatology out-patient appointment and liver ultrasound scan after liver function tests at a routine annual check had shown an alkaline phosphatase eight times the upper limit of normal. Otherwise she complained only of many years of troublesome 'rheumatism'. On examination she was in obvious discomfort. Her distal right thigh and knee were swollen and tender, with overlying hyperaemia, but no knee effusion could be detected clinically. Her temperature was 37 °C. Her facial appearance is shown in the following figure.

1. What is the most likely cause of the pain?
    a) Osteomyelitis
    b) Myeloma
    c) Septic arthritis
    d) Haemarthrosis
    e) Pseudogout
    f) Osteosarcoma
    g) Metastatic carcinoma
    h) Osteoarthritis
    i) Intramuscular haemorrhage

2. Choose the definitive investigation from the following:
    a) Bone biopsy
    b) Blood cultures

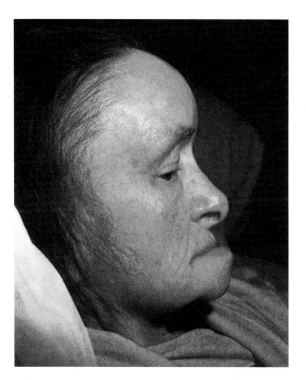

c) Knee aspiration, Gram stain and culture of fluid
d) Knee aspiration and polarizing microscopy of fluid
e) Urine electrophoresis
f) Mammography
g) Bone scintigram
h) Clotting screen

Case 16.4

A 64-year-old lady presented with a one-year history of dysphagia for solids. She had lost 6 kg in weight and was lethargic and more breathless on exercise than usual. She had been diagnosed with Crohn's disease 15 years previously, although this had been quiescent for nearly a decade. Apart from ibuprofen for hip and knee pain she took no other drugs and had no other medical history. The appearance of her hands is shown in the figure at the top of page 132.

1. Which one of the following diagnoses is most likely to explain the dysphagia?
    a) Barrett's oesophagus
    b) Achalasia

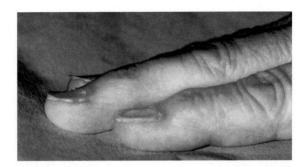

c) Mitral stenosis
d) Oesophageal web
e) Crohn's stricture
f) Systemic sclerosis
g) Oesophageal arteriovenous malformation (AVM)

Case 16.5

A 39-year-old insurance salesman presented with acute abdominal pain and haematuria. He had been well until one month previously, when he noticed increasing swelling of his legs. He commented incidentally that his urine had appeared frothy for some time. On examination his temperature was 37.6 °C. His JVP was not visible, blood pressure was 140/80 mmHg, and there was pitting oedema to the waist. His chest was dull at the right base, with decreased air entry. His left iliac fossa and left loin were markedly tender. Bowel sounds were present, rectal examination was normal, and examination of the genitalia revealed only a right-sided varicocoele.

Hb 12.6 g/dl, white cell count 13.8 × 10⁹/l, Na 132 mmol/l, K 4.3 mmol/l, urea 15.2 mmol/l, creatinine 220 μmol/l, albumin 14 g/l, fasting glucose 4.9 mmol/l. CXR: right pleural effusion. Urinalysis: red cells +++, protein +++.

The plain abdominal radiograph is shown in the figure at the top of page 133.

1. Which cause for the abdominal pain would be at the top of the differential diagnosis?
    a) Nephrolithiasis
    b) Haemorrhage into a renal cyst
    c) Renal vein thrombosis
    d) Constrictive pericarditis
    e) Pyelonephritis
    f) Splenic infarct
    g) Pancreatitis

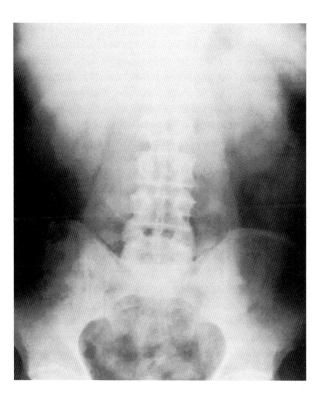

2. What is the most likely underlying diagnosis?
   a) Hyperparathyroidism
   b) Amyloidosis
   c) Polycystic kidney disease
   d) Diabetes
   e) Malaria
   f) Tuberculosis
   g) Membranous glomerulonephritis
   h) Crescentic glomerulonephritis
   i) Paroxysmal nocturnal haemoglobinuria

Case 16.6

A 24-year-old lady was 22 weeks into her second, uncomplicated pregnancy when she began to suffer vaginal bleeding. Her blood pressure was 110/60 mmHg. She had no oedema. Full blood count, electrolytes and uric acid were all normal. The bleeding continued and an ultrasound confirmed premature rupture of her membranes. There were no fetal movements and no fetal heart sounds. Over the next 24 hours she received

3 l of fluid with oxytocin to induce delivery of her missed abortion at the recommended dose of 2–5 mU/min. She failed to deliver but became increasingly drowsy, culminating in a generalized tonic–clonic seizure, to which the RMO was called. On arrival she had recovered. Her blood pressure was 110/60 mmHg and her fingerprick glucose was 7 mmol/l.

1. What is the immediate reason for the seizure?
   a) Pre-eclampsia
   b) Amniotic fluid embolism
   c) Hyponatraemia
   d) Encephalitis
   e) Hypocalcaemia
   f) Meningococcal septicaemia
   g) DIC due to retained dead fetus

Case 16.7

A 28-year-old telephonist developed a tingling feeling in her feet, which ascended her legs over a period of six hours. She found that she was tripping over her toes when walking and had difficulty climbing stairs. She noticed some pain in the middle of her back. One year previously she had developed a right-sided weakness, which resolved in five hours. Two months later she developed a DVT. Investigations at that point confirmed a primary antiphospholipid syndrome with no associated disorder. She was commenced on warfarin. One week prior to the current admission she had been treated with a five-day course of penicillin V for shortness of breath and a cough productive of green sputum. Her GP had noted myringitis. She took no other medications. There was no history of allergies or recent foreign travel. On examination she was afebrile and the myringitis appeared to have cleared up. She had no lymphadenopathy. Higher mental function, cranial nerve and upper limb examinations were normal. Tone was decreased in the lower limbs, with grade 3/5 weakness proximally and 4/5 distally. Biceps and triceps jerk were normal, but knee and ankle jerks were obtainable only with reinforcement. Both plantars were up-going. Vibration sense, proprioception and pain perception were all impaired to a level of T8. Anal tone was lax. The remainder of the examination was normal.

Full blood count, electrolytes, liver function tests and CXR were all normal. ANA, rheumatoid factor, ASOT and TPHA were all negative. CSF: protein 0.68 g/l, five white cells, no organisms.

1. Select the most likely diagnosis from the following list:
   a) Brainstem infarct
   b) Vertebral artery dissection
   c) Epidural haematoma
   d) Multiple sclerosis
   e) Epidural abscess
   f) Anterior spinal artery infarct
   g) Guillain–Barré syndrome

2. It is 6 p.m. and you are based in a hospital with limited out-of-hours imaging capabilities. Which of the following management decisions would you make?
   a) Transfer to observation ward, watch for deterioration, and arrange urgent CT scan of brain for the following morning
   b) Call in consultant radiologist to restart CT scanner and scan brain that evening
   c) Transfer to hospital for MRI brain that evening
   d) Transfer to hospital for MRI spinal cord that evening
   e) Transfer the following morning for MRI brain
   f) Transfer the following morning for MRI spinal cord

Case 16.8

A 46-year-old housewife presented with a three-day history of increasing headache, nausea and vomiting. In her past medical history she had a renal transplant four years previously for polycystic kidney disease. The operation had been a success and the kidney continued to work well. On examination she was febrile but had no rash. She was not drowsy but had mild meningism. A non-tender transplanted kidney was palpable in the right iliac fossa. Examination was otherwise normal.

1. Her CT brain scan (below) shows:
   a) Subarachnoid blood
   b) Dilated lateral ventricles

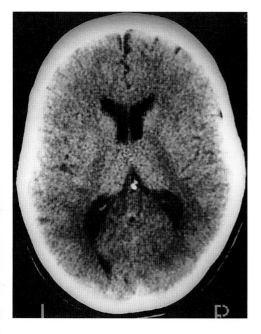
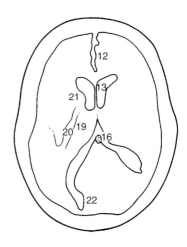

   c) Displaced fourth ventricle
   d) Cerebral aneurysm
   e) Normal scan

Lumbar puncture: 300 white cells, one red cell, 95% lymphocytes, protein 0.64 g/l, glucose 1.2 mmol/l (blood glucose 5.5 mmol/l), no organisms seen on Gram stain or Ziehl–Nielsen stain. Cryptococcal antigen negative.

2. The CSF glucose is:
   a) Normal
   b) Low
   c) High
   d) Normal after correction for lymphocyte count

3. Select from the following the three most likely diagnoses:
   a) Subarachnoid haemorrhage
   b) Subacute hydrocephalus
   c) *Listeria* meningitis
   d) Tuberculous meningitis
   e) Cryptococcal meningitis
   f) Early bacterial meningitis
   g) Viral meningitis
   h) Partially treated bacterial meningitis

Case 16.9

A 63-year-old woman, the wife of a vicar, was admitted because of a confusional state. That morning she had been shopping, driven back home and gone to assist with the flower arranging, but she could not remember what she was supposed to be doing or why she was there. She did not recognize her friends, who thus arranged hospital admission. By the time she reached hospital, several hours later, she appeared to be entirely normal, although she could not remember anything from setting off to the shops to arriving at hospital. Her accompanying friend said her speech and gait were normal in church, with no abnormal movements. She had no past medical history and had displayed no functional deficits prior to that day. There was no history of trauma. Examination was entirely normal.

Full blood count, electrolytes, CXR and ECG were all normal.

1. Select three possible diagnoses from the following:
   a) Hypoglycaemic attack
   b) Arrhythmia
   c) Complex partial epilepsy
   d) Hysterical fugue

  e) Transient ischaemic attack
  f) Transient global amnesia
  g) Post-concussion

2. Choose three investigations from the following that you would carry out:
  a) CT/MRI head
  b) 24-hour cardiac tape
  c) Angiography of vertebral vessels
  d) Blood glucose/48-hour fast
  e) Carotid Doppler
  f) Psychiatric referral
  g) EEG

Case 16.10

A 37-year-old man presented with leg swelling, oedema and hair loss. He had no abdominal pain, nausea or vomiting and had noticed no blood in his stools, although they were sometimes pale. He had no recent foreign travel, no infectious contacts and no relevant past medical or family history. On examination he had dystrophic nails and alopecia totalis. There was no glossitis or stomatitis. He was hyperpigmented. His JVP was not raised and his heart sounds were normal. He had just detectable ascites but marked peripheral oedema. There was no palpable organomegaly.

Hb 10.4 g/dl, MCV 77 fl, white cell count 4.5×10^9/l, platelets 288×10^9/l, urea 2.4 mmol/l, creatinine 67 μmol/l, albumin 26 g/l, ALT 28 U/l. Urine dipstick: normal.

1. What is the diagnosis?
  a) Peutz–Jeghers syndrome
  b) Abetalipoproteinaemia
  c) Cronkhite–Canada syndrome
  d) Polyglandular autoimmune syndrome
  e) Gardner's syndrome
  f) Coeliac disease

Exam 17

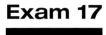

Case 17.1

A 52-year-old woman is referred on account of left foot pain dating from a minor fall some two months before. Radiographs in the accident and emergency department at the time of the injury had failed to reveal any fracture, and rest and simple analgesia had been advised. Despite this, the pain had failed to settle, although weight-bearing was possible. Otherwise, systemically she had been well. Her past history was of hypertension, diabetes diagnosed eight years before and treated with tablets for five years, chronic mild asthma and a cholecystectomy two years before.

Examination of the feet revealed all pulses to be intact, with some evidence of distal symmetrical sensory neuropathy. The left foot was obviously warmer than the right, with distended superficial veins. There was marked tenderness over the medial aspect of the foot. The plain radiograph again failed to show any evidence of fracture. The bone scintigram is shown below:

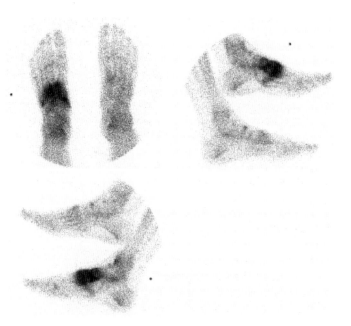

1. What is the likely diagnosis?
   a) Osteomyelitis
   b) Avascular necrosis in tarsal bones
   c) Charcot neuroarthropathy
   d) Reflex sympathetic dystrophy
   e) Metastasis
   f) Non-union of occult fracture

2. What step would you recommend next?
   a) Total contact plaster cast
   b) Bone biopsy and culture
   c) MRI of the right foot
   d) Surgical exploration of the foot and internal fixation
   e) FDG PET imaging of the foot
   f) Chest radiography

Case 17.2

A 28-year-old man underwent a cadaveric renal transplant for renal failure due to Alport's syndrome. Two years later in the review clinic it was noted that his liver function tests had deteriorated progressively. He was otherwise well. He was teetotal and compliant with his medication.

ANA, SMA and LKM antibody testing were negative. Alpha-1 anti-trypsin levels were normal. MCV 102 fl. Serum caeruloplasmin and copper levels were normal. Hepatitis B surface antigen was negative. Anti-hepatitis C antibody was negative. No alcohol detected in blood or urine. Liver biopsy showed an intense lobular infiltrate of mononuclear cells.

1. Which one of the following diagnoses is most consistent with this scenario?
   a) Alcoholic liver disease
   b) Chronic autoimmune hepatitis
   c) Hepatic veno-occlusive disease
   d) Budd–Chiari syndrome
   e) Chronic active hepatitis secondary to hepatitis C reactivation
   f) Chronic active hepatitis secondary to hepatitis B reactivation

2. Which of the following would be diagnostic?
   a) PCR for hepatitis C RNA
   b) PCR for hepatitis B RNA
   c) Hepatic ultrasound with Doppler traces
   d) Trial of increase of the steroid dose
   e) Change of immunosuppression regimen
   f) MRI of the abdomen, with gadolinium enhancement

Case 17.3

A 23-year-old cleaner presented with presyncope after two days of melaena. She had been found to be iron-deficient one year previously, responding to a three-month course of oral supplements. Her current haemoglobin was 7.2 g/dl, with an iron deficiency picture. Her past medical history was unremarkable, although she had never experienced menarche. On examination she was short (1.46 m) and had multiple pigmented naevi on her trunk. Cardiovascular examination revealed a moderate intensity ejection systolic murmur but otherwise normal heart sounds. She was pale, with a postural systolic blood pressure drop of 25 mmHg. No other abnormality was detected.

After transfusion, she was investigated. OGD, barium follow-through and colonoscopy were all normal. Abdominal ultrasonography revealed only an incidental horseshoe kidney. Urology follow-up was arranged. One month later she presented with a further bout of melaena.

1. Choose the single most likely diagnosis from each of the two groups below:
   a) Karyotype 47, XXY
   b) Karyotype 46, XX
   c) Karyotype 46, XY
   d) Karyotype 45, X/46, XX
   e) William's syndrome
   f) Noonan's syndrome
   g) MEN1

   h) Portal hypertensive gastropathy
   i) Enteric angiodysplasia
   j) Meckel's diverticulum
   k) Small-bowel neoplasm
   l) Small-bowel Crohn's disease
   m) Small-bowel ulcers

2. Which of the following is the most appropriate next step?
   a) ^{99m}Tc-pertechnate scan
   b) ^{99m}Tc-tetrofosmin scan
   c) ^{99m}Tc-*sesta*MIBI scan
   d) Laparotomy
   e) Enteric angiography
   f) Abdominal ultrasonography with vascular traces

Case 17.4

A 70-year-old man presented with difficulty rising from chairs and diffuse bone pain, which had gradually developed over three months. Apart from bilateral cataract extractions two years previously, his past medical and drug history was unremarkable. He had bilateral corneal arcus and Dupuytren's contractures. His proximal muscles were weak. Examination was otherwise normal.

Hb 11.2 g/dl, white cell count 8.4×10^9/l, platelets 320×10^9/l, ESR 80 mm/h, Na 137 mmol/l, K 3.0 mmol/l, chloride 110 mmol/l, bicarbonate 15 mmol/l, urea 4.5 mmol/l, creatinine 106 µmol/l, albumin 36 g/l, calcium 2.4 mmol/l, phosphate 0.5 mmol/l, ALP 130 U/l, glucose 4.2 mmol/l, total protein 90 g/l, urate 0.11 mmol/l. Arterial blood gas: pO_2 14.6 kPa, pCO_2 3.2 kPa, pH 7.32. Urine dipstick: glucose +++, protein +++, pH 5.0. Abdominal X-ray: normal.

1. Select two likely diagnoses:
    a) Renal tubular acidosis (RTA) type 2
    b) RTA type 4
    c) RTA type 1
    d) Mixed connective tissue disease
    e) Myeloma
    f) Polymyositis
    g) Diabetic nephropathy
    h) Diabetic amyotrophy
    i) Polymyalgia rheumatica

2. Which one of the following will be one of the next investigations you arrange?
    a) EMG and nerve conduction studies
    b) Bone scintigraphy
    c) Urine electrophoresis
    d) Trial of steroids
    e) Renal biopsy
    f) Oral glucose tolerance test
    g) CK determination

Case 17.5

An 18-year-old student was found to be markedly hypertensive at induction to the local gym, and so he consulted his GP. He drank to excess occasionally, smoked five cigarettes per day and had an unremarkable past medical and family history. He currently felt well. His blood pressure was raised persistently, and thus he was referred to clinic.

On examination his morphology was normal. His pulse was 90/min and regular and blood pressure was 160/110 mmHg in both arms, with no postural drop. The JVP was not visible. His apex beat was forceful but undisplaced. He had normal heart sounds, no abdominal bruits, no organomegaly and no radiofemoral delay. Grade II Keith–Wagener changes were seen on fundoscopy. The remainder of the examination was normal.

Na 140 mmol/l, K 2.9 mmol/l, urea 4.3 mmol/l, creatinine 86 µmol/l, albumin 40 g/l, ALP 86 U/l, arterial pO_2 12.5 kPa, pCO_2 5.8 kPa, bicarbonate 32 mmol/l, pH 7.47, urine dipstick normal, recumbent plasma aldosterone 10 pmol/l (normal: 100–450 pmol/l).

1. Which two of the following top the differential diagnosis?
    a) Glucocorticoid-suppressible hyperaldosteronism
    b) Syndrome of apparent mineralocorticoid excess
    c) Renin-secreting tumour
    d) Hypoaldosteronism
    e) Type IV renal tubular acidosis
    f) Liddle's syndrome
    g) Bartter's syndrome
    h) Gitelman's syndrome
    i) Conn's syndrome

Case 17.6

A 45-year-old woman, the wife of a vicar, developed double vision. When she covered one eye she saw only one image, but this was slightly blurred. By the time she reached hospital two hours later she found that her speech was becoming slurred (which she ascribed to her dry mouth). She had been well until the day of admission. Her past medical history was unremarkable and she took no medications. She was afebrile, with a normal general examination. Higher mental function was intact. Pupils were both 5 mm in diameter and poorly reactive. There was a bilateral partial ptosis, with impaired abduction of both eyes. Corneal reflexes were intact, with normal facial sensation. Speech was nasal in quality, with decreased palatal movement. Tongue movements were impaired, although the mouth was very dry. Grade 4/5 weakness of neck flexion and extension was evident. Limb examination was normal.

1. Suggest two possible diagnoses from the following list:
    a) Diphtheria
    b) Atropine ingestion
    c) Guillain–Barré variant
    d) Tick paralysis
    e) Organophosphate poisoning
    f) Botulism
    g) Shellfish ingestion
    h) Myasthenia gravis
    i) Paralytic rabies
    j) Snake bite

2. Choose one investigation from the following to distinguish these quickly:
    a) Nerve conduction studies
    b) Tensilon test
    c) Lumbar puncture

Case 17.7

A 22-year-old woman sought medical attention on account of menstrual irregularity and problems conceiving. She also admitted to fatigue and regular headaches, which she ascribed to a stressful job. She took no medication. Confrontation testing in clinic suggested a bitemporal lower quadrantanopia.

Full blood count, electrolytes and liver function tests were all normal. LH 2.2 U/l, FSH 1.1 U/l, prolactin 3000 U/l, TSH 1.9 mU/l, free T_3 4 pmol/l (normal: 9–25 pmol/l). An insulin stress test was performed, achieving a minimum blood glucose of 1.6 mmol/l. Further results of the stress test were as follows:

	Basal	Maximal
GH (mU/l)	0.1	0.2
Cortisol (nmol/l)	240	520

1. Which of the following diagnoses best explains these findings?
   a) Prolactin-secreting macroadenoma
   b) Prolactin-secreting microadenoma
   c) Hypothyroidism
   d) Craniopharyngioma
   e) Anterior pituitary sarcoidosis

2. If the diagnosis is confirmed, what is the definitive management most likely to be?
   a) Cabergoline and review
   b) Cabergoline and then surgery
   c) Surgery
   d) Stereotactic radiotherapy
   e) Steroids
   f) Thyroxine

Case 17.8

A 40-year-old man presented with a swollen tender right calf. He was otherwise well and had no relevant past medical or family history. He did not smoke or drink and he took no medications. On examination he was slim and plethoric and had signs consistent with a right above-knee DVT. No other abnormalities were found.

Na 137 mmol/l, K 3.6 mmol/l, urea 4.4 mmol/l, creatinine 77 μmol/l, Hb 22.2 g/dl, MCV 83 fl, PCV 70%, white cell count 5.6×10^9/l, platelets 340×10^9/l, pO_2 14.3 kPa, pCO_2 4.4 kPa.

1. Which two of the following are the most likely diagnoses?
   a) Renal cell carcinoma
   b) Eisenmenger's syndrome
   c) Stress polycythaemia (Gaisböck's syndrome)
   d) Obstructive sleep apnoea
   e) Polycythaemia rubra vera
   f) Von Hippel–Lindau disease
   g) Liver cirrhosis with AV shunting
   h) Chronic myeloid leukaemia

2. Which one of the following investigations will discriminate these two possibilities?
   a) CT head
   b) Leukocyte alkaline phosphatase
   c) CO-Hb determination
   d) ^{51}Cr-red cell scan
   e) Bone marrow trephine

Case 17.9

An 18-year-old student was referred with increasing malaise over three weeks. Her past medical history was unremarkable, although she had not yet undergone menarche. Her breasts had begun to enlarge at age 13. She was taking no medication. She was a keen runner and did not smoke. On examination she was 5′ 10″. (Her parents were 5′ 7″ and 5′ 4″.) She did not look acromegalic or Marfanoid. Breasts and genitalia appeared normal, but axillary and pubic hair were scanty. A right-sided pelvic mass was palpable.

Full blood count and electrolytes: normal. LH 40 U/l, FSH > 50 U/l, plasma 17-β-oestradiol 124 pmol/l (normal: follicular phase 75–260 pmol/l, mid-cycle 370–1470 pmol/l), β-HCG mid-cycle 3000 U/l. Bone age 13.

1. Give two diagnoses on the basis of these findings:
   a) Pregnancy
   b) Turner's syndrome
   c) Pituitary adenoma
   d) Androgen insensitivity syndrome
   e) Ovarian stromal tumour
   f) Hydatidiform mole
   g) Hypothyroidism
   h) Dysgerminoma
   i) Reifenstein syndrome

Case 17.10

A 22-year-old student presented with a three-week history of increasing abdominal pain and abdominal and leg swelling. She felt under the weather but was managing to continue her studies. She reported no fevers or sweats and could remember no infectious contacts. Her past medical history was unremarkable, her only recent foreign travel was to Paris, and the only medication she took was the contraceptive pill. On examination there were no stigmata of chronic liver disease. Her pulse was 80/min and regular, blood pressure was 110/70 mmHg, venous pressure was not elevated, heart sounds were normal and chest was clear. Her abdomen was distended, with tender hepatomegaly (particularly the right lobe) and prominent ascites. There was no splenomegaly. She had marked dependent oedema.

Hb 11.4 g/dl, white cell count 8.5×10^9/l, platelets 338×10^9/l, Na 139 mmol/l, K 3.9 mmol/l, urea 5.6 mmol/l, creatinine 97 μmol/l, albumin 35 g/l, ALT 45 U/l, ALP 160 U/l, bilirubin 19 μmol/l. Urine dipstick: normal.

1. What is the most likely diagnosis?
    a) Portal vein thrombosis
    b) Budd–Chiari syndrome
    c) Intra-abdominal malignancy
    d) Acute hepatitis
    e) Autoimmune liver disease
    f) Restrictive cardiomyopathy

2. Select the definitive investigation from the following:
    a) Echocardiography
    b) Liver biopsy
    c) Ascitic tap and cytology
    d) Liver ultrasonography with Doppler traces
    e) Hepatic venography
    f) Prothrombin time

Exam 18

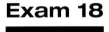

Case 18.1

A 58-year-old alcoholic was referred from casualty. He was inebriated so no history was available, although he did appear to be indicating epigastric discomfort and was obviously in some distress. On examination he had stigmata of chronic liver disease but was neither icteric nor obviously encephalopathic. He was afebrile but tachycardic at 130/min, with an irregularly irregular rhythm and blood pressure of 110/50 mmHg. His chest was clear. There was some epigastric tenderness but no guarding and normal bowel sounds. A detail of his chest radiograph is shown below:

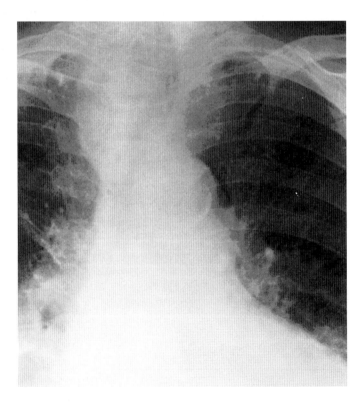

He was admitted for observation and a few hours later he had deteriorated. He was now febrile at 38.7 °C and had a pulse rate of 150/min and blood pressure of 80/40 mmHg. There was dullness to percussion at the left base, with decreased air entry on auscultation, and hyper-resonance to percussion in the left upper zone, also with decreased air entry.

1. What is the diagnosis?
    a) Friedlander's pneumonia (*Klebsiella*)
    b) Acute pancreatitis
    c) Evolving lung/cardiac contusion
    d) Boerhaave's syndrome
    e) Aortic dissection
    f) Post-primary TB with pericardial involvement

Case 18.2

A 47-year-old businessman was referred to neurology clinic because he kept tripping over his toes. The problem had begun about three months ago with numbness of his right foot and a floppy ankle, with the left foot following suit a few weeks later. On direct questioning he had some pain in both wrists and elbows, which he related to recurrence of an old whiplash injury following a road traffic accident in France, when his spleen was removed. On examination his hands were white and cold. There was no arthritis and no upper-limb neurological signs. He did, however, have signs consistent with a lower-limb sensorimotor neuropathy.

His legs are shown below:

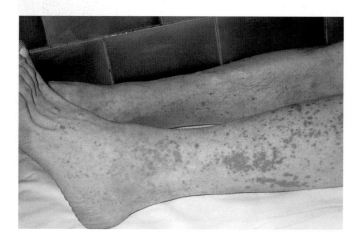

Hb 13.7 g/dl, white cell count 13.3 × 10⁹/l, platelets 430 × 10⁹/l, clotting studies normal, urea 4.5 mmol/l, creatinine 98 μmol/l, ALT 55 U/l, ALP 80 U/l, bilirubin 9 μmol/l, rheumatoid factor 1/640. ANA and ANCA negative. HIV, VDRL and TPHA negative. Blood cultures: no growth. CXR and CT abdomen normal.

1. What is the most likely diagnosis?
   a) Mixed essential cryoglobulinaemia
   b) Type II cryoglobulinaemia
   c) SLE
   d) Rheumatoid arthritis

2. Select two investigations from the following list that you would carry out:
   a) Immunoglobulins
   b) Hepatitis C serology
   c) HBV/EBV/CMV serology
   d) Nerve conduction studies
   e) Sural nerve biopsy

Case 18.3

A 23-year-old man had taken two days of a five-day course of co-amoxiclav for presumed sinusitis with a purulent discharge from a blocked right nostril and postnasal drip when he became photophobic. He had no previous medical history and there was no reason to suspect immunosuppression. On examination he was febrile at 38.2 °C, with tenderness over the right maxillary and frontal sinuses and purulent discharge visible in the right nares. Neurological examination was normal. An enhanced CT scan of his head confirmed the sinusitis. The intracranial cavity was normal. On re-examination 24 hours later he now had grade 4 left-sided weakness.

1. Select three possible diagnoses from the following list:
   a) Left frontal lobe abscess
   b) Right frontal lobe abscess
   c) Cortical venous infarction
   d) Subdural empyema
   e) Hydrocephalus with medullary coning
   f) Meningitis
   g) Normal-pressure hydrocephalus

Case 18.4

A 16-year-old boy was treated by his GP with amoxicillin for a respiratory tract infection featuring cough and wheeze. His infection settled promptly, but he was left with intermittent niggly abdominal pain and occasional nausea and non-bloody diarrhoea. One month later he presented as an emergency with increasingly severe abdominal pain, constipation, nausea and vomiting. Examination revealed a distended abdomen with generalized tenderness and guarding. Bowel sounds were tympanic, hernial orifices were normal and his rectum was empty. Plain abdominal radiography showed dilated loops of small bowel.

Hb 14.7 g/dl, white cell count 12.4×10^9/l (neutrophils 65%, lymphocytes 27%), platelets 245×10^9/l, K 3.2 mmol/l, urea 8.6 mmol/l.

1. What is the most likely diagnosis?
    a) Mesenteric adenitis
    b) Crohn's disease
    c) Meckel's diverticulum
    d) Toxocariasis
    e) Ascariasis
    f) Trichuriasis
    g) Appendicitis

Case 18.5

A 22-year-old man was admitted directly to ICU after suffering a cardiac arrest at a local gym. Fortunately, automated defibrillation had been available. The defibrillator had diagnosed ventricular fibrillation and had administered a shock. The patient was not known to have any previous medical history and had been well recently. Transthoracic echocardiography in ICU showed a structurally normal heart but with depressed systolic function, presumed consequent upon the arrest.

1. Consider the following list of diagnoses:
    a) Wolff–Parkinson–White syndrome
    b) Athlete's heart
    c) Lown–Ganong–Levine syndrome
    d) Romano–Ward syndrome
    e) Brugada syndrome
    f) Hypertrophic cardiomyopathy
    g) Anomalous coronary anatomy
    h) Myocarditis
    i) Arrhythmogenic right ventricular dysplasia

For each of the figures on page 150, select a single option from the list above.

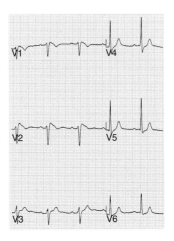

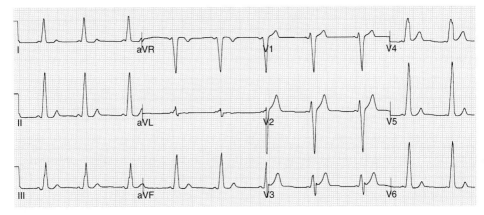

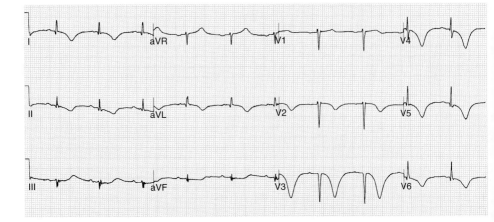

Case 18.6

A 26-year-old management consultant attended her first insurance medical. She was fit and well. Her past medical history was unremarkable except for removal of her tonsils and adenoids at age eight. She considered her family healthy, although she recalled her father having a surgical scar on his neck. She took no drugs, including the contraceptive pill. She did not smoke and she drank alcohol only occasionally. Examination was entirely normal.

Urea 3.4 mmol/l, creatinine 66 μmol/l, Na 138 mmol/l, K 4.2 mmol/l, corrected calcium 2.8 mmol/l on repeated uncuffed samples, phosphate 0.8 mmol/l, albumin 36 g/l, PTH 3.9 pmol/l (normal: <0.9–5.4 pmol/l). Serum ACE, TSH, Igs and CXR: all normal. 24-hour urine calcium 2.4 mmol (normal: 2.5–7.5 mmol).

1. What is the next step?
   a) *Sesta*MIBI nuclear imaging of the neck
   b) Creatinine clearance, DXA of bone, and renal ultrasonography
   c) Surgical referral
   d) Six-monthly serum calcium
   e) 25-hydroxy-vitamin D
   f) Screen *ret* proto-oncogene
   g) Gut hormone profile and catecholamines

Case 18.7

A 68-year-old man presented with a six-month history of progressive clumsiness of his right hand and gait disturbance. On examination he had an expressionless facies and he walked with a slow, shuffling gait. He had limb rigidity and bradykinesia. A presumptive diagnosis of Parkinson's disease was made. He was commenced on Madopar 125® (co-beneldopa) four times daily.

1. He is unable to tolerate his medication because of nausea. Which two of the following measures would you recommend?
   a) Take co-beneldopa before food
   b) Take co-beneldopa after food
   c) Take co-beneldopa standing up and do not sit down for 30 minutes
   d) Co-administer prochlorperazine
   e) Co-administer metoclopramide
   f) Co-administer domperidone

These measures solve the problem and he successfully increases his dose to 1 × Madopar 125 at 7 a.m., noon, 5 p.m. and 10 p.m. This controls his symptoms for approximately six months, but he then begins to find he becomes stiff from about an hour before the next dose is due.

2. What would you recommend?
   a) Increase dose to 1.5 × Madopar 125 at 7 a.m., noon, 5 p.m. and 10 p.m.
   b) Increase dose to 1 × Madopar 125 at 7 a.m., 11 a.m., 3 p.m., 7 p.m. and 11 p.m.
   c) Change to a controlled-release Madopar preparation, 1 × Madopar CR at 7 a.m., noon, 5 p.m. and 10 p.m.

Six months later he is admitted for assessment because of increasing confusion. This is variable but particularly prominent at night. He also reports frequent visual hallucinations.

3. Which of the following measures would be the most appropriate?
   a) Decrease dose of Madopar
   b) Keep Madopar the same and introduce haloperidol
   c) Keep Madopar the same and introduce droperidol
   d) Keep Madopar the same and introduce chlorpromazine

This measure works for a few months, but his condition then deteriorates, with increasing falls and memory loss.

4. What diagnosis would you now consider to be most likely?
   a) Wilson's disease
   b) Multiple system atrophy
   c) Normal-pressure hydrocephalus
   d) Dementia with Lewy bodies
   e) Severe Parkinson's disease

Case 18.8

A 40-year-old man presented with a 36-hour history of increasing drowsiness. He said he had contracted flu five days previously and had been laid up in bed and off food since then. He had been an insulin-dependent diabetic for the past 20 years and had recently had laser therapy to both eyes. He had no neuropathy or nephropathy detectable at his last clinic visit. He took a twice-daily mixed insulin and an ACE inhibitor. He was teetotal. On examination he was dehydrated and hyperventilating. He was afebrile but drowsy. Pan-retinal photocoagulation scars were seen but there was no focal neurology. The remainder of the examination was normal.

Finger-prick glucose 9.5 mmol/l, Hb 13.5 g/dl, white cell count 14.3×10^9/l (80% neutrophils), platelets 458×10^9/l, Na 136 mmol/l, K 5.7 mmol/l, chloride 95 mmol/l, urea 10.4 mmol/l, creatinine 180 μmol/l, blood glucose 10.8 mmol/l, bicarbonate 8 mmol/l, lactate 2.9 mmol/l (normal: 0.6–1.7 mmol/l), pH 7.06, pO_2 15.4 kPa, pCO_2 1.8 kPa. Clotting studies, liver function tests, CXR and ECG: all normal. Blood cultures: no growth. Urine dipstick: ketones +++. Urine microscopy: all normal. Paracetamol and salicylate levels: negative.

1. What is the diagnosis?
   a) Diabetic ketoacidosis (DKA)
   b) Type A lactic acidosis
   c) Type B lactic acidosis
   d) D lactate acidosis
   e) Ethylene glycol toxicity

Case 18.9

A 60-year-old man presented with a hoarse voice. He gave a five-year history of seropositive rheumatoid arthritis. He had presented initially with hand and wrist arthritis together with subcutaneous nodules and was treated with a NSAID. Over the past year his disease had become increasingly severe, with ankle and knee involvement rendering him almost immobile. He was prescribed sulphasalazine, but this had to be stopped because of a rash. He was converted to penicillamine. The rash cleared up and his arthritis seemed to be getting better, but he then noticed that his voice was steadily going hoarse. On examination he had signs of a symmetrical deforming arthropathy with volar subluxation of the metacarpophalangeal joints and ulnar deviation of the fingers. Early swan-neck deformities were evident on several fingers. Elbow and knee joints appeared normal. There was some forefoot deformity. There was no tenderness at any joint and no evidence of any synovitis. No subcutaneous nodules were palpable. On neurological examination he had decreased abduction of his left eye, together with a lack of both inferomedial and superior movements of his right eye. There was a partial ptosis of the right eyelid. Palatal movement was markedly decreased, resulting in nasal speech. The remainder of the examination was normal.

Full blood count, electrolytes, liver function tests, ECG and CXR: all normal.

1. What is the diagnosis?
   a) Guillain–Barré syndrome
   b) Active rheumatoid arthritis
   c) Myasthenia gravis
   d) Grave's disease
   e) SLE
   f) Botulism

2. Select two investigations from the following list that you would carry out:
   a) Vital capacity
   b) Anti-acetylcholine receptor antibody titre
   c) CT chest
   d) Thyroid function tests
   e) Gastric lavage
   f) Autoantibodies

Case 18.10

A 20-year-old man with acute promyelocytic leukaemia was placed on allopurinol prior to his first cycle of chemotherapy. His pre-chemotherapy bloods were as follows: Na 128 mmol/l, K 7.8 mmol/l, chloride 100 mmol/l, urea 5.4 mmol/l, creatinine 80 mmol/l.

The technician said that there was no haemolysis, the correct tube had been used and the sample was labelled as having been taken that day. Urine dipstick was normal. The blood was not taken from the drip arm.

1. Suggest two possible diagnoses.

Exam 19

███████████

Case 19.1

A 38-year-old Moroccan kebab vendor presented to casualty with difficulty in swallowing his saliva. He commented that his neck and jaw muscles had, on several occasions, gone into spasm for 15–30 minutes, although on examination in casualty only his masseters appeared stiff, manifesting as a difficulty in jaw-opening. His teeth and throat appeared normal. There was no meningism. Chovstek's and Trousseau's signs were negative. One week previously he had cut his finger while gardening. Two days before he had four loose bowel motions, which settled that day. The night before admission he had been given some tablets to take at a nightclub. Further details were not forthcoming, except that he had not been abroad for two years. Full blood count, electrolytes, calcium, phosphate and blood gases were all normal.

1.   Suggest from the following three possible diagnoses:
   a)   Hypocalcaemia
   b)   Rabies
   c)   Tetanus
   d)   Ecstasy reaction
   e)   Hysteria
   f)   Hypomagnesaemia
   g)   Guillain–Barré syndrome
   h)   Botulism
   i)   Strychnine poisoning
   j)   Meningitis

Case 19.2

An 18-year-old student presented with blurring of his vision when walking downstairs. There were no other symptoms. He had no past medical history and had reached his childhood milestones normally. Not sporty at school, he had now taken to rowing, although he often developed pain in his head and neck at full slide. On examination he appeared normal but had a low hairline. Visual fields were full, with normal fundi. Eye movements were full, but with downbeat nystagmus on looking downwards. A decrease in pinprick sensation was apparent on the right-hand side of his face. His palatal movement and tongue appeared normal. Limb examination was normal. He had an ataxic gait.

1. Where is the anatomical site of the pathology?
   a) Foramen magnum
   b) Medulla
   c) Pons
   d) Midbrain
   e) Occipital cortex
   f) Brainstem

2. What is the likely diagnosis?
   a) Platybasia
   b) Syringomyelia with Chiari malformation
   c) Basilar invagination
   d) Klippel–Feil syndrome
   e) Base-of-skull tumour

Case 19.3

A 36-year-old man presented with a two-day history of chills, muscle aches, sweating and frontal headaches. He had been off his food and felt very tired. He had suffered no cough, chest pain, abdominal symptoms or dysuria. He had been well previously, apart from mild asthma, and a fractured femur and emergency splenectomy after a motorcycle crash at the age of 19. He did not smoke, he drank around 20 units of alcohol per week, and he had a sedentary job. His only recent travel had been a camping holiday on the Massachusetts coast (north-east USA). On direct questioning, he said that he had been bitten on several occasions by both mosquitoes and ticks, but he remembered no rashes.

On examination his temperature was 40 °C, his pulse rate was 115/min, and his blood pressure was 120/80 mmHg. He appeared unwell and icteric, without stigmata of chronic liver disease. Auscultation of the heart was normal, while abdominal examination revealed the scar of his previous surgery and two-finger hepatomegaly. His chest was clear, there were no enlarged lymph nodes, and neither meningism nor focal neurology could be demonstrated. There were no rashes.

Hb 11.2 g/dl, white cell count 9.8×10^9/l, platelets 40×10^9/l, clotting normal. Na 135 mM, K 4.3 mM, urea 7.8 mM, creatinine 135 μM, albumin 35 g/l, ALP 180 U/l, ALT 54 U/l, bilirubin 48 μM, haptoglobin undetectable. Urinalysis: blood ++. CXR: normal. Two sets of blood cultures were negative.

Over the next 48 hours his condition deteriorated despite treatment with cefotaxime and erythromycin. The haemoglobin dropped to 8 g/dl and acute renal failure developed. He was admitted to ICU.

1. Which of the following diagnoses best explains the above scenario?
   a) Lyme disease
   b) Tick-borne relapsing fever

  c) Rocky Mountain spotted fever
  d) *Plasmodium falciparum* malaria
  e) *Plasmodium vivax* malaria
  f) Babesiosis

2. One day later, a Giemsa-stained blood film was examined, which was said by the technician on call to show 20% infection with single intra-erythrocyte ring forms. In the light of this, which of the above diagnoses would you now favour?

3. Which definitive treatment would you recommend?
  a) High-dose penicillin
  b) Intravenous quinine
  c) Intravenous quinine and clindamycin
  d) Penicillin and doxycycline
  e) Doxycycline
  f) Quinine then primaquine

Case 19.4

A 65-year-old man presented with a two-month history of increasing lethargy, weight loss and tingling fingers. He had no previous medical history, although he smoked 20 cigarettes per day and he had a sister with diabetes. On examination he was thin. His pulse was 80/min, blood pressure was 120/80 mmHg and JVP was not raised. His chest was clear. There was peripheral oedema to his thighs. Decreased sensation was detected in his thumb, index and middle fingers bilaterally with +ve Tinel's sign.

Hb 11.7 g/dl, white cell count 6.5×10^9/l, platelets 280×10^9/l, urea 6.0 mmol/l, creatinine 110 μmol/l, albumin 22 g/l, random glucose 7.1 mmol/l. Urine dipstick: protein ++++. Rheumatoid factor, ANA and anti-dsDNA antibodies all negative.

1. What is the most likely underlying diagnosis?
  a) Occult carcinoma
  b) Small-vessel vasculitis
  c) Diabetes mellitus
  d) AL amyloidosis
  e) AA amyloidosis
  f) Heavy metal poisoning

Case 19.5

A 20-year-old car mechanic presented to casualty when a piece of machinery fell on him and broke his arm. The uncomplicated left radial fracture was splinted with a plaster of Paris cast. He was advised to visit his GP on account of raised blood pressure detected by the routine nursing observations. On two follow-up visits to his GP, when he was not in pain his blood pressure was found to be raised persistently at 160/100 mmHg. His past medical and family history was unremarkable, and he took no drugs or herbal remedies. He drank 10 units of alcohol per week. No primary cause for the hypertension was suggested by a thorough examination; nor was there any evidence of end-organ damage.

Na 134 mmol/l, K 5.7 mmol/l, urea 5.1 mmol/l, creatinine 105 μmol/l, albumin 40 g/l, calcium 2.4 mmol/l, phosphate 1.0 mmol/l. Full blood count, clotting, ECG and CXR: all normal. Urine dipstick: normal. 24-hour urine Na excretion: 15 mmol/24 h (normal: 100–250 mmol/24 h). Recumbent plasma aldosterone: 20 pmol/l (normal: 100–450 pmol/l).

1. What is the diagnosis?
    a) Hypoaldosteronism
    b) Addison's disease
    c) Gordon's syndrome
    d) Type IV renal tubular acidosis (RTA)
    e) Liquorice excess
    f) Liddle's syndrome

Case 19.6

A 26-year-old nurse presented with malaise, sweatiness and palpitations. She had no past medical history. Her mother had Grave's disease. On examination she was sweaty, with a fine tremor of the outstretched hands. There was a small, non-tender goitre with no bruit. Examination of the eyes revealed lid lag and lid retraction. There was no lymphadenopathy. Her pulse was 100/min and regular.

Free T$_4$ 35 pmol/l (normal: 9–25 pmol/l), TSH < 0.04 mU/l, ESR 28 mm/h.
The result of ^{99m}Tc-scintigraphy is shown here:

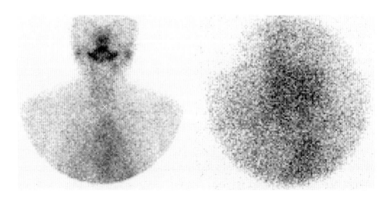

1. Select the two most likely diagnoses in order of probability:
   a) De Quervain's thyroiditis
   b) Grave's disease
   c) Autoimmune thyroiditis
   d) Riedl's thyroiditis
   e) Single autonomous thyroid nodule
   f) Syndrome of resistance to thyroid hormone
   g) Toxic nodular goitre
   h) Struma ovarii

2. What treatment would you suggest for the most likely diagnosis?
   a) Corticosteroids and propranolol
   b) Propylthiouracil and propranolol
   c) Carbimazole and propranolol
   d) Oral iodine
   e) Propranolol only

Case 19.7

An 18-year-old man presented with a two-month history of irritability, sweatiness and breast enlargement. His past medical history was unremarkable. He smoked five cigarettes per day, drank alcohol occasionally, but took no drugs. On examination he was clinically mildly thyrotoxic, with a small goitre, and there was obvious gynae-comastia. He appeared unable to follow the examiner's finger upwards on testing of eye movements. Examination was otherwise normal.

Full blood count, electrolytes and liver function tests: all normal. LH 25 U/l (normal: 3–8 U/l), FSH 5.0 U/l (normal: 0.5–5.0 U/l), free T_4 36 pmol/l (normal: 9–25 pmol/l), TSH 0.1 mU/l (normal: 0.5–5 mU/l), testosterone 60 nmol/l (normal: 9–42 nmol/l), 17-β-oestradiol 638 pmol/l (normal: 220 pmol/l).

1. What is the most likely diagnosis?
   a) LH-secreting pituitary adenoma
   b) Testosterone self-administration
   c) Leydig cell tumour of testis
   d) Grave's disease
   e) Teratoma with cerebral metastases
   f) Pinealoma

Case 19.8

A 36-year-old man of Mediterranean appearance presented with haematemesis and melaena. He did not speak any English and thus it was difficult to elicit any further information. On examination he was pale, with cool peripheries. His pulse was 120/min. His blood pressure was 120/80 mmHg when lying down and 100/60 mmHg when sitting. His heart sounds were normal and his chest was clear. There was a surgical scar in the left upper quadrant and a 5-cm palpable liver. Surgical scars were also found overlying his right and left hip and left knee.

Hb 8.4 g/dl, white cell count 4.2×10^9/l, platelets 290×10^9/l, Na 144 mmol/l, K 4.1 mmol/l, urea 6.4 mmol/l, creatinine 104 μmol/l, ALT 45 U/l, total acid phosphatase 15 U/l (normal: 1–5 U/l), serum ACE 98 U/l (normal: 21–54 U/l). OGD revealed bleeding varices.

1. What is the likely underlying diagnosis?
   a) Sarcoidosis
   b) Pompe's disease
   c) Beta-thalassaemia
   d) Gaucher's disease
   e) Alcoholism
   f) Familial Mediterranean fever

2. Select two treatments from the following that may alleviate the underlying problem:
   a) Bone marrow allografting
   b) Liver transplantation
   c) Abstinence from alcohol
   d) Colchicine
   e) High-protein diet
   f) Desferrioxamine
   g) Corticosteroids
   h) Glucocerebrosidase enzyme replacement
   i) Acid α-glucosidase enzyme replacement

Case 19.9

A 30-year-old lady presented with recurrent episodes of presyncope. Six weeks previously she had suffered a swollen painful right index finger. She could remember no trauma. There was no relevant family history. She had immigrated from Somalia five years previously and had recently completed a course of chloroquine and Paludrine® (proguanil) following a trip to Uganda. She was taking no other medications and took no herbal preparations. She had not had any tick bites. Her only symptom on systems enquiry was a long-standing cough productive of white sputum. She smoked 10 cigarettes per day but consumed no alcohol. On examination her blood pressure was 120/80 mmHg with no postural drop. Her pulse rate was 80/min and regular, with JVP raised to 4 cm. Her apex beat was displaced to the sixth intercostal space in the anterior axillary line and was volume-loaded. An apical third heart sound and occasional basal crepitations were audible. Her ankles were swollen. The remainder of her examination was normal.

Full blood count and electrolytes: normal. Bilirubin 23 μmol/l, ALT 55 U/l, ALP 170 U/l, calcium 2.7 mmol/l, phosphate 1.0 mmol/l, albumin 35 g/l. Rheumatoid factor, ANA and anti-dsDNA: all negative. HIV antibody: negative. Tuberculin test (100TU): no reaction. Urine dipstick and microscopy: normal. ECG: prolonged PR interval and right bundle branch block. Sputum: Gram stain and Ziehl–Nielsen stain negative. Angiogram: global decrease in systolic function, all chambers dilated, coronary arteries normal.

1. What is the most likely diagnosis?
    a) Familial transthyretin-associated amyloidosis
    b) Lymphoma
    c) Sarcoidosis
    d) Myocarditis
    e) Chloroquine-induced dilated cardiomyopathy
    f) Tuberculosis

2. Select the most useful diagnostic imaging modality from the following:
    a) Indium-labelled white cell scan
    b) Gallium 67 scintigram
    c) Serum amyloid precursor scan
    d) MIBI scan
    e) ^{99m}Tc scintigram
    f) Cardiac MRI

Case 19.10

A 44-year-old man presented with fever, myalgia, painful testes, and a three-month history of weight loss. On examination he was febrile at 38.2 °C, with a pulse rate of 130/min, blood pressure of 180/110 mmHg and normal heart sounds. The remainder of the examination was normal, apart from tender testes.

Hb 10.3 g/dl, white cell count 14.7 × 10^9/l (80% neutrophils), platelets 440 × 10^9/l. Film: normochromic, normocytic anaemia. Electrolytes, ECG and CXR: all normal. Urine dipstick: blood and protein.

The following day he deteriorated, with severe abdominal pain and vomiting. His abdomen was diffusely tender, with marked guarding. Bowel sounds were absent. Infarcted small bowel was resected at surgery. ANA, rheumatoid factor, anti-dsDNA, ANCA and anticardiolipin antibodies were sent, but all were negative.

1. Select the two most likely diagnoses from the following:
    a) Wegener's granulomatosis
    b) Churg–Strauss syndrome

   c) Microscopic polyangiitis (mPA)
   d) Polyarteritis nodosa (PAN)
   e) Mumps
   f) Paroxysmal nocturnal haemoglobinuria
   g) Infective endocarditis
   h) Takayasu's arteritis
   i) Cholesterol emboli

2. How will you confirm the diagnosis?
   a) Testicular biopsy
   b) Renal biopsy
   c) Histology of resected bowel
   d) Angiography
   e) Magnetic resonance angiography (MRA)
   f) Serology
   g) Ham's test

Exam 20

███████

Case 20.1

A 47-year-old farmer's assistant presented to the neurologists with memory loss. His clinic notes were thick due to eight years of seeing a rheumatologist with episodic seronegative arthritis affecting wrists, ankles, knees and elbows. On direct questioning he admitted to loose, offensive stools over the past six months but not to any abdominal or chest pain, rash, eye problems or ulcers. On examination he was pigmented, with small lymph nodes palpable in the cervical chain, axillae and inguinal regions. His temperature was 37.7 °C. Examination was otherwise normal, except for a generalized impairment of higher mental function. Rheumatoid factor, ANA, TPHA and HIV were all negative. Thyroid function, B12, folate and thiamine levels were all normal.

1. What is the diagnosis?
   a) Limbic encephalitis
   b) Whipple's disease
   c) Coeliac disease
   d) Behçet's syndrome
   e) Polyarteritis nodosa
   f) Familial Mediterranean fever
   g) Reiter's syndrome
   h) Thiamine deficiency

Case 20.2

A 63-year-old man was referred from the vascular surgeons. For the previous three years he had suffered pain in his legs on walking. Initially only in his left buttock at half a mile, with time it had come to involve both buttocks at progressively shorter distances and was associated with tingling radiating down the back of his legs. His pain always disappeared within minutes on rest or on leaning forwards. He was a non-smoker with no past medical history. His erections were normal. Examination at rest was normal. All peripheral pulses were present with no bruits. He had been referred because aortography was entirely normal.

1. Select the single most likely diagnosis from the following:
   a) Takayasu's arteritis
   b) Lumbar plexopathy
   c) Lumbar disc prolapse
   d) Atherosclerosis of distal spinal arteries
   e) Intraspinal tumour
   f) Retroperitoneal fibrosis
   g) Lumbar stenosis syndrome

Case 20.3

A 32-year-old chemist presented with a four-month history of lethargy, weight loss and night sweats. He had also latterly suffered several episodes of bloodstained diarrhoea. He had emigrated from Bangladesh 11 years previously. On examination he was febrile and mildly tender in the right iliac fossa, with a palpable spleen tip.

Hb 10.2 g/dl, white cell count 9.2 × 109/l. Electrolytes, liver function, CXR, AXR and urinalysis were all normal. Bone marrow and liver biopsies were normal on histology and culture. Mantoux at one in 10 000 was negative. Barium follow-through revealed multiple shallow ulcers and several discrete strictures in the terminal ileum. Colonoscopy showed inflammation of the proximal colon, although the caecum could not be reached. Biopsy showed only non-specific inflammatory changes.

1. Which two of the following are top of the differential diagnosis?
   a) Tuberculosis
   b) Ileal adenocarcinoma
   c) *Yersinia* infection
   d) T-cell lymphoma of the terminal ileum
   e) Behçet's disease
   f) Whipple's disease
   g) *Salmonella* typhlitis
   h) Gastrinoma
   i) Amoebic dysentery
   j) Crohn's disease

2. Choose the next step from the following list:
   a) Trial of corticosteroids
   b) Trial of mesalazine
   c) Trial of anti-tuberculous therapy
   d) Laparotomy and biopsy
   e) Abdominal CT imaging

Case 20.4

A 36-year-old man had suffered bouts of renal colic several times per year for the past 15 years. An attack would normally subside spontaneously, often with the passage of small, spiculated stones. During a particularly severe attack, he was forced to attend casualty. This attack settled after a pethidine injection. The casualty doctor ordered an abdominal X-ray, which is shown below:

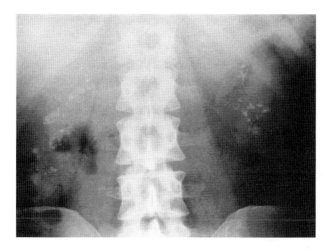

In the follow-up clinic, he reported that apart from the attacks of colic he was otherwise well. He had no past medical or family history and took no drugs. Examination was entirely normal.

Full blood count, electrolytes, liver function tests, calcium, phosphate, urate, TSH, blood pH, CXR and hand X-ray were all normal. 24-hour urine calcium, phosphate, oxalate, urate and protein excretion were all normal.

1. What is the most likely underlying diagnosis?
    a) Medullary cystic disease
    b) Polycystic kidney disease
    c) Analgesic nephropathy
    d) Nephrocalcinosis
    e) Schistosomiasis
    f) Medullary sponge kidney
    g) Sarcoidosis

2. What would be your next investigation?
    a) Abdominal ultrasonography
    b) Locker search
    c) Renal biopsy

    d) Intravenous pyelogram
    e) MAG3 renogram

Case 20.5

A 46-year-old salesman presented to clinic with a two-month history of increasing fatigue and weight loss. His only other symptom of note had been vague abdominal pains. His presentation to the doctor was precipitated by a marked increase in lethargy and shortness of breath over the preceding week. There was no melaena. On examination he was thin, pale and jaundiced. Xanthelasma were evident, as were palmar erythema, bilateral Dupuytren's contractures and two spider naevi.

There was no encephalopathy. Pulse was 90/min and regular. Blood pressure was 120/70 mmHg when lying down and 100/60 mmHg when standing. Heart sounds were normal and the JVP was not visible. A 1 cm, smooth, non-tender, non-pulsatile liver was palpable. There was no other organomegaly. Nystagmus was elicitable on lateral gaze. The fundal appearance is shown below:

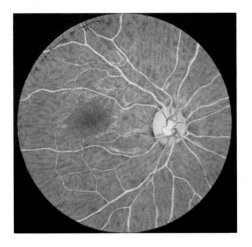

Hb 8.4 g/dl, white cell count 8.3 × 10⁹/l, platelets 130 × 10⁹/l, MCV 105 fl. Film: spherocytes, macrocytes, reticulocytes (12%). INR 1.3. Na 131 mmol/l, K 4.6 mmol/l, urea 4.4 mmol/l, creatinine 62 μmol/l, albumin 30 g/l, calcium 2.3 mmol/l, phosphate 0.8 mmol/l, bilirubin 90 μmol/l, ALT 270 U/l, GGT 170 U/l, ALP 240 U/l. Hepatitis B surface antigen and hepatitis C antibody both negative. Urine dipstick: blood.

1.   Choose the two diagnoses from the following that are most likely to explain these findings:
    a) Alcoholic liver disease
    b) Wilson's disease

c) Haemochromatosis
d) Primary biliary cirrhosis (PBC)
e) Zieve's syndrome
f) Hereditary spherocytosis
g) Pancreatic carcinoma
h) Evans syndrome
i) Myelodysplasia

Case 20.6

A 60-year-old lady presented with a six-month history of weight loss and diarrhoea. She had no nausea, vomiting or abdominal pain, but she would pass frequent, smelly stools. There was no blood admixed. She had begun to feel increasingly weak and lethargic, although she had no other specific symptoms to report. In her past medical history she had a nasal polypectomy eight years previously. She took no medications, smoked 20 cigarettes per day and drank alcohol socially. She was thin and pale, with peripheral oedema, but examination was otherwise normal.

Hb 9.2 g/dl, white cell count $6.4 \times 10^9/l$, platelets $440 \times 10^9/l$, calcium 2.0 mmol/l, albumin 22 g/l, ALT 18 U/l, Fe 10 μmol/l, B12 130 ng/l (normal: 150–750 ng/l), serum folate 9.2 nmol/l (normal: 4.8–6.4 nmol/l). Urine dipstick: normal. Abdominal X-ray: multiple fluid levels. Jejunal biopsy: mild, non-specific inflammation.

1. What is the most likely diagnosis?
   a) Jejunal diverticulosis
   b) Small-bowel obstruction
   c) Crohn's disease
   d) Heavy-chain disease
   e) Giardiasis
   f) Coeliac disease
   g) Whipple's disease
   h) Small-bowel lymphoma

2. Choose two investigations from the following to confirm your diagnosis:
   a) Barium study of small bowel
   b) Hydrogen breath test
   c) Urea breath test
   d) Duodenal biopsy
   e) Faecal fat excretion
   f) White cell scan
   g) Microscopy of stool for ova, cysts and parasites
   h) Laparotomy
   i) Antiendomysial antibodies

Case 20.7

A 45-year-old spinster presented with increasing lethargy, depression and weight gain. She smoked 10 cigarettes per day and drank 30 units of alcohol per week. On examination she appeared Cushingoid. There were no stigmata of chronic liver disease.

Cortisol: 9 a.m. 800 nmol/l, midnight 780 nmol/l, ACTH 9 a.m. 60 ng/l, midnight 45 ng/l.

9 a.m. cortisol after dexamethasone 0.5 mg six-hourly for 48 hours was 90 nmol/l.

1. Which one or more of the following diagnoses are consistent with these data?
   a) Pseudo-Cushing's syndrome
   b) Adrenal adenoma
   c) Adrenal carcinoma
   d) Micronodular adrenal hyperplasia
   e) Pituitary adenoma
   f) Bronchial carcinoid
   g) Surreptitious glucocorticoid self-administration

2. Which two of the following tests would be reasonable next steps?
   a) CRH stimulation test
   b) Glucagon stimulation test
   c) High-resolution CT imaging of the chest
   d) Overnight dexamethasone suppression test
   e) Bilateral inferior petrosal sinus sampling (BIPSS)
   f) Bilateral adrenal vein sampling
   g) Selenocholesterol scintigraphy

Case 20.8

A 54-year-old Italian solicitor was admitted in a coma. He was unable to give any history but his secretary said that the patient, apart from being very tired at work, had been well before going on holiday two weeks previously and was under no obvious psychological stress. He took occasional ibuprofen for what the GP had diagnosed as gout in his hands and knees, and he was on a diabetic diet. On examination he had a GCS of 3/15 and lay with extensor posturing, symmetrical brisk reflexes and up-going plantars.

Finger-prick glucose was found to be 2.4 mmol/l and so 30 ml of 50% dextrose was given intravenously. This failed to have a significant effect on the conscious level.

Hb 11.6 g/dl, platelets 100×10^9/l, Na 133 mmol/l, K 3.2 mmol/l, urea 1.1 mmol/l, creatinine 60 μmol/l, glucose 3.9 mmol/l, chloride 99 mmol/l, HCO_3 11 mmol/l. Paracetamol undetectable. CT head normal. CSF: three white cells, six red cells, no organisms. Arterial PaO_2 13.2 kPa, $PaCO_2$ 4.1 kPa, pH 7.19.

1. Select the most likely diagnoses from the following:
   a) Insulinoma
   b) Addison's disease
   c) Covert use of oral hypoglycaemic agents
   d) Cerebral malaria
   e) Herpes simplex encephalitis
   f) Diabetic ketoacidosis
   g) Aspirin overdose
   h) Haemochromatosis

Case 20.9

A 30-year-old nurse presented with episodic leg weakness and lightheadedness. She would often sweat and be aware of her heart pounding and felt very frightened when this occurred. Friends noted her to become very pale during such episodes. Attacks occurred at any time of day, with no obvious precipitants. She was otherwise well, apart from occasional diarrhoea, with no past medical or family history. She denied any drug-taking. She smoked 20 cigarettes per day and was a social alcohol drinker. Examination showed blood pressure to be 140/95 mmHg when lying down and 115/85 mmHg on standing. Otherwise, no abnormality could be found.

Hb 17.4 g/dl, white cell count 5.5×10^9/l, platelets 230×10^9/l, haematocrit 0.61, Na 144 mmol/l, K 4.3 mmol/l, urea 3.4 mmol/l, creatinine 66 μmol/l, glucose 7.8 mmol/l, albumin 38 g/l, ALT 27 U/l, calcium 2.8 mmol/l, phosphate 0.9 mmol/l, PT 13 s (normal: 10–12 s). Chest radiography was normal. The ECG is shown below:

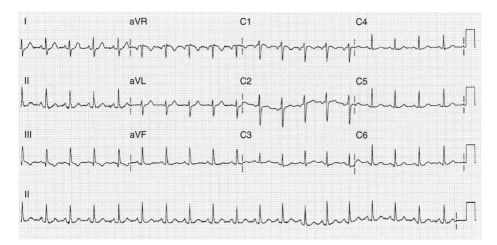

1. Select the two most likely diagnoses from the following list:
   a) Addison's disease
   b) Lown–Ganong–Levine syndrome

   c) Parathyroid adenoma
   d) Insulinoma
   e) MEN1
   f) Phaeochromocytoma
   g) Long QT syndrome
   h) Parathyroid hyperplasia
   i) Surreptitious insulin abuse
   j) Carcinoid syndrome

2. Choose the most important next step:
   a) 72-hour fast with glucose and C-peptide measurements
   b) Short synacthen test
   c) 24-hour ECG
   d) Electrophysiological studies
   e) PTH levels
   f) Abdominal CT with contrast
   g) Pituitary MRI
   h) Fasting gastrin and prolactin levels
   i) Urine or plasma catecholamines

Case 20.10

A four-year-old girl underwent cardiac catheterization:

	Pressure (mmHg)	O_2 saturation
IVC	12	55
RA	12/0	54
RV	104/8	57
PA	18/10	63
LV	108/9	90
Aorta	105/5	82

1. Which of the following diagnoses best fits the data?
   a) Ebstein's anomaly
   b) Pulmonary stenosis
   c) Patent ductus arteriosus
   d) Fallot's tetralogy
   e) Atrial septal defect

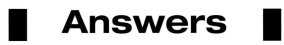 # Answers

Exam 1

■■■■■■■■

Case 1.1

1. d
2. a, b, f

The answer is in the pulmonary function tests (PFTs). The PEFR is abnormally low for the FEV_1. However, the normal ranges are not needed to reach the diagnosis. Just calculate the FEV_1 (in ml) to PEFR (in l/min) ratio. This is termed the Empey index. The ratio is less than 10 in normal subjects and in those with lung disease intrinsically affecting the airways, e.g. asthma and COAD. A ratio greater than 10 occurs with upper-airway obstruction. This reflects the fact that PEFR is largely effort-dependent and is affected disproportionately by a proximal obstruction. In contrast, the FEV_1 reflects more the effort-independent phase of expiration, which is affected less by a proximal obstruction. In patients with sleep-related upper-airway resistance syndrome, the obstruction is episodic and related to position and level of consciousness. An alert patient would not show this pattern of PFT abnormalities.

During a forced inspiration, negative pressure develops throughout the airways. This negative pressure becomes much greater if there is a proximal obstruction through which the air needs to be sucked. The air surrounding the airways outside the pleura (extrathoracic) remains at atmospheric pressure; thus, if the airways are mobile (e.g. if the obstruction is due to bilateral vocal cord palsy), they will collapse, causing a flat inspiratory flow limb (Figure (b) below). During expiration, the positive pressure forcing the air out of the lungs also holds the mobile obstruction apart, and the expiratory loop therefore appears relatively normal. In contrast, if the obstruction fixes the airways in place (e.g. a tracheal tumour), then both the expiratory and inspiratory phases will be decreased (Figure (c) below). The reduction in expiratory flow rates is most marked at the higher flow rates, causing a blunted peak to the expiratory flow curve (i.e. the PEFR) with a relatively normal later curve (i.e. the FEV_1 is less affected). The noisy breathing (stridor) but clear chest is classical. A similar picture could result from a poorly co-operative patient not trying very hard or from respiratory muscle weakness. The best confirmatory test is a flow-volume loop. The CXR may show a mediastinal mass, although this may be small and may be confused with vascular lesions, particularly if asymmetrical. A CT is therefore very useful. A goitre would be high on the differential diagnosis of fixed extrathoracic airflow obstruction – multinodular goitres are by far the most common. One would only proceed to bronchoscopy having excluded a goitre and other mediastinal masses.

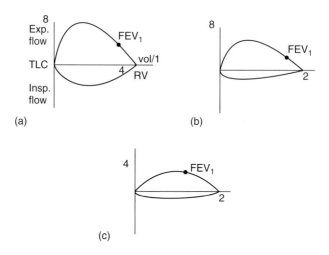

Flow-volume loops: (a) normal; (b) variable extrathoracic obstruction (maximum inspiration more limited than maximum expiration); (c) fixed extrathoracic obstruction (marked limitation of both inspiration and expiration).

Causes of localized upper-airway obstruction include:

- Tracheal stenosis, e.g. post-intubation
- Tracheal abnormalities, e.g. tracheomalacia
- Recurrent laryngeal nerve palsy
- Oedema, e.g. allergy, angioneurotic oedema, smoke inhalation
- Infection, e.g. croup, epiglottitis, retropharyngeal abscess, tonsillitis
- Lymphadenopathy
- Tumours, e.g. thymoma
- Intrathoracic goitre
- Aneurysm
- Tracheal disease, e.g. amyloidosis, granulomatous diseases

Case 1.2

1. d
2. b

The chest film shows multiple lesions consistent with septic emboli. This scenario is classical for Lemierre's disease, a variety of necrobacillosis. Necrobacillosis is infection by *Fusobacterium necrophorum* at various sites, with resultant tissue necrosis and abscess formation. Necrobacillosis affecting the throat is termed Lemierre's disease. It usually affects the young, who classically suffer a severe sore throat followed by painful cervical lymphadenopathy and septic thrombophlebitis of the tonsillar vein, spreading to the internal jugular vein. Metastatic abscesses develop, particularly in the lungs. *Fusobacteria* respond slowly to benzylpenicillin and metronidazole. Abscesses must be sought and drained.

Vincent's angina is a necrotizing periodontitis and gingivitis caused by mixed organisms, including anaerobes, while Ludwig's angina is a rapidly spreading sublingual and submandibular cellulitis, often consequent upon an infected molar. The same agents and principles of treatment apply.

Case 1.3

1. f
2. h

Half of all patients with hepatic granulomata present with a pyrexia of unknown origin. Out of the long list of infective causes, TB is the commonest; thus, a trial of anti-tuberculous therapy is justified if it cannot be excluded confidently. Of note, atypical mycobacteria may be responsible and are often resistant to standard regimens. Cat-scratch fever may cause isolated granulomata, but *Bartonella henselae* should be seen with the Warthin–Starry stain. Incriminated drugs – in this case, the classical agent tolbutamide – should be stopped. After a reasonable initial search for one of the causes listed below, a trial of steroids would then be pragmatic and appropriate, although further investigation may subsequently be required should this fail:

- Infections:
  - bacteria: TB, leprosy, *Brucella*, cat-scratch fever, *Listeria*, *Yersinia*, Whipple's disease
  - spirochetes
  - fungi: histoplasmosis, cryptococcosis, candidiasis, coccidioidomycosis
  - rickettsia: Q fever
  - parasites: *Toxocara*, schistosomiasis, leishmaniasis, visceral larva migrans
  - AIDS
- Drugs: beryllium, allopurinol, antiepileptics, clofibrate, sulphonamides, sulphonylureas, diazepam, contraceptive pill, *p*-aminosalicylic acid
- Carcinoma and lymphoma
- Sarcoidosis
- Immune deficiency: hypogammaglobulinaemia, chronic granulomatous disease
- Autoimmune disease: PBC, ulcerative colitis, Crohn's, SLE, PMR, giant cell arteritis
- BCG vaccine
- Idiopathic

Case 1.4

1. e

Several diseases may cause endocrine dysfunction and dilated cardiomyopathy, but the only one to cause specific macroscopic changes that would enable the surgeon to make the diagnosis at operation is haemochromatosis: the heart appears brown. (You can assume, quite reasonably, that the surgeon did not make the diagnosis preoperatively.) Haemochromatosis is among the commonest inherited conditions in northern Europe, with a carrier frequency of around one in seven for one of the two common point mutations in the HFE gene. Its penetrance is, however, very variable. Joint involvement most commonly starts with the second and third metacarpophalyngeal joints, involving large joints later, and around half of cases have evidence of chondrocalcinosis.

Case 1.5

1. a
2. a, d, h

Cerebellar signs are ipsilateral. Gait ataxia localizes to the vermis. Cerebellar haemangioblastomas often cause a polycythaemia. Although only rarely part of the classical von Hippel–Lindau syndrome, mutations in the VHL gene are increasingly recognized in patients with isolated haemangioblastomas. In this case, the family history of renal cell carcinoma raises the diagnostic possibility enough for a correct MRCP answer. VHL is a dominantly inherited cancer syndrome due to a mutation in VHL, a tumour suppresser gene. Other haemangioblastomas may occur elsewhere in the CNS. It is associated with retinal angiomatous malformations and cystic lesions in the pancreas, kidney and adrenals, which may also develop haemangioblastomas. Renal cell carcinomas may also develop. Patients need to be screened regularly for tumour development and progression. Polycythaemia may be due to either a haemangioblastoma of the cerebellum or a hypernephroma. It is also associated with phaeochromocytomas.

Lowe's (oculo-cerebro-renal) syndrome is a rare X-linked recessive condition causing cataracts from birth, along with mental retardation and renal failure. It is beyond the scope of MRCP and was included only as a red herring.

Case 1.6

1. d
2. c
3. b

The history of acute left iliac fossa pain followed by bloody diarrhoea in an arteri-opath with a probable history of mesenteric angina makes ischaemic colitis the most likely diagnosis. The poor anastomotic channels make the splenic flexure and descending colon particularly prone to vascular occlusion. The radiograph shows irregular, thickened mucosa ('thumbprinting') along the whole transverse colon and proximal descending colon. The most useful investigation is a barium enema. Acute thumbprinting is characteristic, although any grossly swollen bowel wall can thumbprint, and less specific ulceration may develop subsequently. Although abdominal X-ray may also show thumbprinting, as well as loss of haustrations and narrowing, with intramural gas in cases of infarction, it is much less sensitive. Sigmoidoscopy and stool microscopy will help exclude other causes of colitis. Colonoscopy risks perforating the ischaemic segment acutely. It may show a blue swollen mucosa with a normal rectum. Angiography is helpful only occasionally. Rigler's sign refers to the visible presence of gas on both sides of the bowel wall on a supine film, a sign of pneumoperitoneum. An example is shown below:

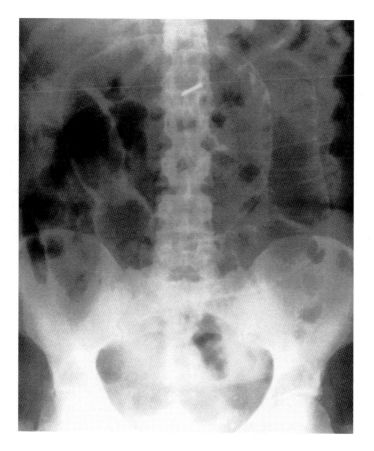

Case 1.7

1. d
2. a

Xanthine and urate stones are radiolucent. The other stones are radio-opaque, although cystine and magnesium ammonium phosphate stones tend to be fainter than calcium oxalate and phosphate stones. Oxalate stones are spiky; cystine stones are pale yellow and crystalline. The normal serum and urine calcium levels and, excepting the stone, normal IVP make a high-calcium stone unlikely. (The issue is sometimes complicated, e.g. when a cystine stone acts as a nucleus for the formation of a calcium phosphate stone.) Cystinuria is autosomal recessive and is the commonest cause of nephrolithiasis in childhood, while comprising 1–2% of all renal calculi. The absorption of the dibasic acids cystine, ornithine, arginine and lysine from the proximal tubule and gut is defective. Cystine is the least soluble and thus gives rise to (pathognomonic) hexagonal crystals. Addition of sodium nitroprusside produces a cherry red colour and is particularly important in patients (up to half) with mixed stones. Treatment is with a high fluid intake, urine alkalinization (but if too alkaline, then there is increased risk of calcium stones) and penicillamine.

Cystinosis is a quite discrete multisystem disorder caused by a deficiency of a lysosomal carrier protein. Ocular problems are prominent.

Case 1.8

1. a
2. c
3. a

Rhabdomyolysis is a common cause of acute renal failure, particularly on ITU. It is often picked up late because muscle pain or history of muscle injury may be absent. Thus, the diagnosis needs to be considered in any patient whose dipstick is positive for blood. An absence of red blood cells on microscopy confirms the diagnosis. This may be quicker and cheaper than a specific myoglobin assay. Typical biochemistry is high phosphate and potassium, with low calcium. The muscle enzymes CK, aldolase, AST and LDH may be very high. The myoglobin is less likely to crystallize in the presence of alkaline urine, so many units will give regular small aliquots of alkali until the urine pH is raised, providing a good urine output is maintained. Stopping the NSAID would be appropriate in any acute renal failure but is not a specific management step.

Associations of rhabdomyolysis include:

- Epilepsy
- Any cause of coma or immobility

- Drug addiction
- Malignant hyperpyrexia
- Prolonged exercise
- Myositis
- Infection (particularly viral)
- McArdle's syndrome
- Alcohol
- Carbon monoxide poisoning
- Overdose, e.g. MAOI
- Fibrates and HMGCoA inhibitors
- Glue sniffing
- Phaeochromocytoma
- Surgery
- Snake bite

Case 1.9

1. b

Note that CT scans will not usually pick up brainstem infarcts. However, there are no intrinsic brainstem signs to suggest this as the diagnosis. Together with the extensor posturing, a diffuse cortical pathology seems likely, i.e. an encephalopathy. Causes include encephalitis (less likely given the lack of pyrexia, focal signs, neck stiffness and seizure activity), subarachnoid haemorrhage or meningitis (we would expect some neck stiffness in a patient able to respond to pain), and anoxia or metabolic insults. In an alcoholic with normal electrolytes, the most likely diagnosis is therefore hepatic encephalopathy.

Case 1.10

1. b

Distinguish between classical CJD, a sporadic, rapidly progressive dementia, and vCJD. Particular features of CJD may be mimicked by lithium toxicity, metabolic encephalopathies, paraneoplastic encephalitides (e.g. limbic encephalitis), inflammatory disease, AIDS dementia, Alzheimer's disease and Dementia with Lewy Bodies. However, a rapidly progressive dementia, together with myoclonus, akinetic mutism, cortical blindness, pyramidal or extrapyramidal signs, and in particular an abnormal startle response, strongly suggest CJD, making this the best answer. EEG shows pseudoperiodic sharp waves.

  In contrast, in vCJD, early psychiatric features are prominent, followed by ataxia, involuntary movements and cognitive impairment. Patients tend to be younger than those with classical CJD, and disease duration is longer (vCJD: mean age of death 29, mean duration of illness 14 months). In vCJD, EEGs do not show the classical changes seen in classical CJD, 50% have a positive 14-3-3 immunoassay and over 70% have bilateral pulvinar high signal intensity on MRI. All cases are homozygous for methionine at codon 129 of the prion protein gene.

Antidepressants in overdose may cause myoclonic movements but would not explain the pyramidal signs. Huntington's chorea is more insidious with more prominent choreiform movements, although younger sufferers may be akinetic, i.e. parkinsonian (Westphal variant).

Exam 2

██████████

Case 2.1

1. a
2. d

This patient is likely to be atopic (nasal spray) and asthmatic (wheezy from teens). Prospective studies suggest that 7–14% of such patients fulfil diagnostic criteria for ABPA. Its natural history is progression from corticosteroid-dependent disease to irreversible fibrosis. This patient has an eosinophilia (sum the differential). The CXR is typical. Serum precipitins are only weakly positive, unlike those in aspergilloma, which are strongly positive, while total IgE and *Aspergillus*-specific IgE are both likely to be raised. Eradication is difficult and usually temporary, so therapy is directed at controlling the inflammatory response with steroids. There is also small-scale trial evidence that addition of itraconazole improves outcomes without increased toxicity.

CXR changes include:

- Transient non-segmental shadowing (eosinophilic pneumonia), often perihilar and upper zones
- Tubular shadows and band shadows from bronchial obstruction and dilation
- Tram lines following sputum expectoration
- Upper-zone fibrosis

Case 2.2

1. d
2. c

Invasive disease from mucor-like fungi causes paranasal destruction and lung and skin necrosis and may disseminate. Diabetic ketoacidosis is associated particularly with rhinocerebral involvement. It also occurs in other immunocompromised states. A cellulitis involving *S. aureus*, *S. pyogenes* and anaerobes could evolve into a necrotizing fasciitis, but the clinical picture with only slight erythema but necrotic turbinate makes that less likely. Wegener's needs to be considered in the differential but is not most likely in this classical clinical context. Treatment is urgent debridement and high-dose amphotericin. The syndrome may be due to a variety of organisms, some are relatively easy to culture but others of which are not. Serology is also negative, therefore the diagnosis is often confirmed on histology. Other rare life-threatening infections seen particularly in patients with poorly controlled diabetes are emphysematous cholecystitis, emphysematous pyelonephritis and malignant otitis externa.

Case 2.3

1. b, e, g

The imperative in this case is to consider and take all reasonable steps to rule out an early postoperative infection, either in or around the prosthesis or in the wound/sternum. Serial blood cultures have already been negative, but further blood cultures, transoesophageal echocardiography, and possibly imaging of the sternum and surrounding areas may be appropriate. However, the most likely diagnosis is post-pericardiotomy or Dressler's syndrome. The post-pericardiotomy syndrome occurs one week to two months postoperatively and consists of pericardial and pleuritic pains and an effusion with a raised ESR. Prospective series have suggested it occurs in 7–19% of patients undergoing cardiac surgery. It is understood incompletely, but it is thought to result from exposure of cryptic myocardial antigens and generally remits swiftly with aspirin or NSAIDs, although corticosteroids may also be used. Occasionally, it can lead to pericardial tamponade, or pericardial constriction in the longer term, and can recur over periods up to two years.

Although a progressive AV conduction block may be a critical sign of aortic root infection, first-degree heart block may also occur in the context of calcific aortic valve disease, as in this case. Serial monitoring would be important. The post-transfusion syndrome is thought to represent transfusion-acquired viral infection, most commonly CMV, but the risk of this has been reduced enormously by the recent practice of leucodepletion of donor blood.

Other miscellaneous causes of pericardial effusions to remember include:

- Haematoma
- Talc or cellulose granuloma
- Vasculitis
- Mycobacteria (often tuberculin test negative)

Case 2.4

1. d
2. c

Visceral leishmaniasis is a widespread and burgeoning disease and is epidemic in, eastern India. People who are malnourished or HIV-positive are particularly susceptible. Most cases of visceral leishmaniasis are subclinical. Indian patients often become hyperpigmented. Those reaching doctors often feel well despite obvious clinical signs. IgG is markedly increased, IgM less so (note the large total protein-albumin difference here). Diagnosis is by serology or biopsy. The spleen gives the highest sensitivity but is prone to haemorrhage, and with high parasitic burden bone marrow aspiration is likely to give the diagnosis. Cell-mediated immunity to *Leishmania* in visceral disease is undetectable, and so intradermal Leishmanin testing is futile. A hypopigmented macular rash may develop after one to two years in patients who recover spontaneously (post-kala-azar dermal leishmaniasis). Treatment is with pentavalent antimonals, pentamidine or amphotericin B (liposomal form is less toxic).

A lymphoma would be unlikely to cause this degree of splenomegaly and lymphadenopathy without much systemic illness. Acute myeloblastic leukaemia would be unlikely to cause such marked splenomegaly and blast cells would usually be seen, even in a pancytopoenic presentation. The lymphadenopathy is a useful pointer away from malaria syndromes. The spleen is very large for *Brucella* and schistosomiasis would not lead to fever and lymphadenopathy.

Case 2.5

1. c

This is the mother of all family trees. Daughters of males are not affected but 50% of the children of these daughters are affected. These children can be of either sex. Thus, the gene is inactivated when passed through the male line and reactivated when passed through a subsequent female line. This is called genomic imprinting. It could equally well be that only males activate the gene. The Angelman and Prader–Willi syndromes are the best examples of this. In the Prader–Willi syndrome, the paternally transmitted allele is silenced, whereas in Angelman's syndrome the maternally transmitted allele is silenced.

Case 2.6

1. a
2. a

Bile salt malabsorption from terminal ileal resection can occur with a normal B_{12} level. Diarrhoea is often worst in the morning on release of the overnight gallbladder store. Diarrhoea will cease on fasting, when no bile salts are released. Depletion of the enterohepatic circulation may result in steatorrhoea (which would be worse later in the day). Some centres offer testing with the radiolabelled bile salt analogue homotaurocholic acid. Gamma scanning allows the fate of this (absorption versus excretion) to be analysed. Cholestyramine is effective treatment (particularly when faecal fat excretion is less than 20 g/day) and may aid diagnosis in the absence of nuclear medicine. There are no signs of disease activity to suggest Crohn's disease. Generalized malabsorption of nutrients, salt and water is unlikely after such a short resection. The serum folate is often elevated in bacterial overgrowth.

Case 2.7

1. a

In an analogous way to neurology, the first step is to localize the site of the disorder. The glycosuria, mild hypokalaemia and low serum urate point to proximal renal tubule dysfunction. The normal concentrating ability suggests the distal tubule is unaffected. Protein loss is usually mild (1–2 g/24 h) and non-selective, with β_2-microglobulin levels prominent (although non-specific). Glomerular loss may be much greater but is predominantly albumin. The clue to the cause of the pathology is the occupational history. Cadmium is used in smelting. Acute inhalation may lead to acute pneumonitis, chronic inhalation to tubular damage, emphysema and osteomalacia. A prominent industrial outbreak occurred in Japan in 1946, where itai-itai disease, or multiple painful fractures, was caused by cadmium-induced osteomalacia. Full marks are given just for saying heavy-metal poisoning. (Note: African with vitiligo and nephrotic syndrome – ?mercury-containing, skin-lightening cream used.)

Causes of proximal tubulopathy include:

- Inborn errors of metabolism
- Heavy metals
- Old tetracycline
- Familial
- Hyperparathyroidism
- Hypokalaemia
- Myeloma
- Wilson's disease

Case 2.8

1. e
2. e
3. h

The features described are those of a hyperviscosity syndrome: visual and neurological disturbance, bleeding and thrombosis. Retinal vessels may appear tortuous, progressing to a string-of-sausages appearance and then the production of haemorrhages and exudates. A frank central retinal vein occlusion may also occur from the hyperviscosity. Bleeding may be due to paraprotein coating the platelets. Platelet function tests will be abnormal. Macroglobulinaemia is particularly likely to cause hyperviscosity on account of IgM production. Lymphadenopathy and hepatosplenomegaly are usually, but not always, present at presentation. The IgM may present with features of a cryoglobulin, such as Raynaud's phenomenon and small-vessel vasculitis. Renal failure is uncommon and there are no lytic lesions. Immunoparesis increases susceptibility to infection. Note: intrinsic fever (from IL6 production) is rare. It is usually due to infection. Plasma viscosity is an important acute investigation as plasmapheresis may be indicated as an emergency. Hyperviscosity with IgG myeloma usually occurs only at very high protein concentrations.

Case 2.9

1. a, c, f
2. a, b, d, g

Note the question asks for causes of muscle weakness, not any possible diagnosis, e.g. diabetes. The main differential is that of a raised MCV and muscle weakness. Osteomalacia is very common in elderly people and in Asians. It may present with diffuse pain or immobility from weakness. The raised MCV reflects folate deficiency. In a patient with possible autoimmune disease myasthenia should always be considered, but here it does not link in all the facts. Note that the development of hypothyroidism is a common cause of increasing weakness in myasthenics. This lady has a raised glucose. This does not explain the MCV but may cause proximal weakness, although diabetic amyotrophy is usually painful and asymmetric and is due to nerve rather than muscle pathology. Polymyositis would not explain the raised MCV. It is often painless. Limb girdle dystrophy presents in the second and third decades or rarely in middle age. Dystrophia myotonica would explain the weakness and diabetes, but there are none of the facial characteristics and there is no family history.

Case 2.10

1. d

Attempts to force this combination of several common conditions into a multiglandular endocrinopathy should be resisted! This is a classical setting for late dumping syndrome: rapid gastric emptying leads to a surge in postprandial glycaemia; resulting insulin secretion overshoots, leading to symptomatic hypoglycaemia 90–180 minutes after eating (early dumping is an osmotic phenomenon occurring much earlier) Prolonged oral glucose tolerance tests have been much criticized for their poor sensitivity in spontaneous postprandial symptoms, but in this more concrete scenario early hyperglycaemia followed by significant hypoglycaemia (<2.5 mM) would be diagnostic if occurring with symptoms. Treatment is frequent, small meals with a reduced carbohydrate content. Acarbose, an alpha-glucosidase inhibitor, has also been used with great success in small-scale studies, although flatulence may be a distressing side effect.

Gastric surgery may also reveal latent coeliac disease or hypolactasia, which should be sought if diarrhoea is the main symptom.

Exam 3

Case 3.1

1. d
2. b

The clinical history, radiographic evidence of left upper lobe collapse (raised left hemidiaphragm, 'veiled' appearance of left lung), fluoroscopic evidence of left phrenic nerve palsy and subsequent deterioration make left lingular carcinoma with cardiac tamponade most likely. In this case there is also some right lower lobe consolidation. Pulmonary embolism occurring in the context of a carcinoma cannot, however, be ruled out. All signs elicitable are not always given.

Case 3.2

1. b
2. c

A wide range of conditions such as community-acquired infection, bronchiolitis obliterans organizing pneumonia and PCP could present with this picture, with a deterioration to ARDS. However, hantavirus infection is known to be associated particularly with New Mexico, Colorado, Utah and Arizona. The animal reservoir is in rats and mice, and it produces a diffuse capillary leak syndrome in the lungs of young adults. Some people die from the acute disease, although recovery may be complete. Hantavirus infection in Europe and Asia tends to produce a pulmonary-renal syndrome, with prominent extrapulmonary symptoms in addition. Ribavirin probably aids recovery.

Both *Coccidiodes immitis* and *Histoplasma capsulatum* have very well-known distribution patterns in the southern USA. However, both tend to produce much milder or chronic illnesses that would not fit with this picture.

Case 3.3

1. c
2. e

The clinical history is consistent with acute haemolysis. The circumstantial leap that is helpful is to realize that this student is likely to have just started taking anti-malarial prophylaxis, with the attendant risk of haemolysis in G6PD-deficient individuals. This makes G6PD deficiency most likely in the absence of other information. Many G6PD-deficient patients will have had neonatal jaundice, typically on days two to three. Some have chronic low-grade haemolysis and present with gallstones and splenomegaly. Acute attacks are precipitated by drugs, infection or broad (fava) beans, with a time lag of hours to days. The dark urine is due to haemoglobinuria. During an attack, the most G6PD-deficient red cells may be selectively haemolysed, with a resultant falsely normal G6PD assay in the post-haemolytic phase. Favism is particularly dramatic, with fever, abdominal pain, diarrhoea, vomiting, splenomegaly and, rarely, high-output cardiac failure or hypovolaemic shock. The haemolysis is highly specific to broad (fava) beans. Diagnosis is by red-cell G6PD assay (not serum).

Case 3.4

1. f
2. a, b

In a young patient with appropriate exposure, amoebic abscesses are far more likely than metastatic anaerobic abscesses. Young patients are more likely to present acutely. With a history of less than 10 days, 50% will have multiple abscesses. Beyond 10 days, 80% have a single abscess in the right lobe. Five to ten per cent of patients will have negative serology, in which case it should be repeated after one week. There is often no history of dysentery, and stool analysis in the absence of diarrhoea is of little value. Aspiration of lesions is not routinely useful, even for large abscesses, unless they fail to resolve, they are at risk of rupture, or in cases of diagnostic doubt. Slow resolution with metronidazole is the norm.

Case 3.5

1. b

Always think about renal tubular acidosis when given chloride and bicarbonate values. Wilson's disease may present in many different ways on account of its multi-system pathology, e.g. with fulminant hepatic failure, with acute haemolysis, with tubular damage or with a movement disorder. The signs of liver disease may not be present and the Kayser–Fleischer rings may not be visible to the naked eye.

Possible presentations of Wilson's disease include:

• Cirrhosis with portal hypertension
• Fulminant hepatic failure

- Any movement disorder
- Psychiatric disturbance
- Polyarthritis
- Endocrine disturbance
- Intravascular haemolysis

Case 3.6

1. g
2. d
3. b

Hepatic adenomas are often an asymptomatic chance finding unless their growth is being driven by pregnancy or exogenous oestrogen. The tumours are highly vascular and so should not be biopsied. Liver function tests and AFP are usually normal. Half present with an acute abdomen and shock from a sudden bleed into the tumour or peritoneum. Diagnosis often employs a range of modalities, including MRI, ultrasonography, CT, angiography and ^{99m}Tc-scintigraphy (there are no macrophages in the adenoma, and so an absent signal is seen). Surgery is sometimes required.

The contraceptive pill is also associated with intrahepatic cholestasis, gallstones and the Budd–Chiari syndrome. None of these explains the shock. Herbal remedies could contain lead and result in abdominal pain, but this would not explain the palpable liver or shock. Likewise, acute cholecystitis and amoebiasis might lead to septic shock, but not hypovolaemic shock with acute anaemia. Acute intermittent porphyria may cause sudden abdominal pain and hypotension from autonomic instability but not anaemia.

Case 3.7

1. a

This patient has evidence of renal disease from childhood, with impaired concentrating ability, i.e. medullary pathology. In contrast, the uraemic symptoms appear to be relatively recent, supported by the relatively advanced bone age. Salt wasting was prominent. The skeletal survey showed signs of rickets, renal osteodystrophy and hyperparathyroidism. Medullary cystic disease is an inherited tubulointerstitial nephropathy, with early corticomedullary and intramedullary cysts. Hence, the initial symptoms are those of a concentrating defect. The kidney later becomes shrunken and scarred, with eventual uraemia. It is the cause of 15% of cases of end-stage renal failure in children. Management would include adequate sodium intake, phosphate binders, iron replenishment and erythropoietin, 1-alpha-hydroxylated vitamin D preparations, and plans for transplantation. The disease does not recur after transplantation.

Reflux nephropathy and chronic pyelonephritis would result in an abnormal IVP, while medullary sponge kidney presents most commonly with urinary calculi or haematuria in later life. Autosomal recessive polycystic kidney disease is often a severe disease presenting early in childhood. It is associated strongly with hepatic fibrosis.

Case 3.8

1. e
2. d, e

The osmolality is very high. $(Na + K) \times 2 + urea + glucose \approx$ serum osmolality. Therefore, the glucose is around 45 mmol/l (there is no reason to suspect the presence of any further osmotically active substance in this case). The diagnosis of DKA then falls into place. The radiograph shows gas both in the gallbladder and its wall, suggesting that it is infected with a gas-forming organism; this is a well-recognized and potentially fatal complication in diabetes. Similar emphysematous infections may affect other organs in diabetes, e.g. the bladder. The bilirubin would be higher in cholangitis and this would not explain the mass. Further essential investigations include blood cultures, arterial blood gas determination, urinalysis, and imaging of the biliary tree and gallbladder with ultrasound or CT. Treatment is as for DKA, plus parenteral antibiotics with anaerobe cover. Surgery is necessary either acutely or on recovery. Other noteworthy causes of acalculous cholecystitis include CMV and *Cryptosporidium* infection in AIDS, and polyarteritis nodosum.

Case 3.9

1. c, e

Calculate the anion gap. This leaves you with the small differential of a normal anion gap hypokalaemic acidosis: renal tubular acidosis, acetazolamide therapy, pancreatic fistulae, severe diarrhoea, ureterosigmoidostomy, hydrochloric acid, ammonium chloride or arginine hydrochloride ingestion. Working through each of these possibilities, it is relatively easy to reach the diagnosis with which all the facts fit. Ureterosigmoidoscopy is an old-fashioned urinary diversion operation for cases of malignant obstruction that is used rarely on account of the side effects. A severe acidosis may result, particularly when urine is not emptied from the bowel regularly. Frequent urinary tract infections and the development of osteomalacia are also seen. There is also a high risk of colonic carcinoma developing adjacent to the ureters.

Case 3.10

1. b
2. b, e, h

The carcinoid syndrome develops in gut tumours only if there are hepatic metastases. It may also occur with primary bronchial (the bronchus is derived from the embryonic foregut), ovarian or testicular carcinoid. Left-sided valve lesions are said to occur with bronchial carcinoid or in the presence of a right-to-left shunt. Pellagra, arthritis and sclerotic bone metastases are seen occasionally. ACTH is sometimes secreted, resulting in Cushing's syndrome (with a much more indolent course than that seen with small-cell carcinoma of the lung, when the classical features of Cushing's syndrome rarely have time to develop). Numerous modalities may be employed in the search for a small tumour, including CT, MRI, octreotide or MIBG scintigraphy, arteriography and selective venous sampling. In the presence of metastases, the mainstay of specific treatment is octreotide, but management should ideally occur in a specialist centre with expert knowledge of the relative merits in individual cases of surgery, chemotherapy, palliative embolization of metastases and trial therapies such as radio-octreotide.

The differential diagnosis of flushing also includes:

- Medullary thyroid carcinoma
- Phaeochromocytoma
- Diabetes (N.B. autonomic neuropathy, chlorpropamide)
- Menopause
- Mastocytosis
- Diencephalic seizures
- Drugs (e.g. niacin, calcium channel blockers, disulfiram)

Exam 4

Case 4.1

1. a, f
2. c, e

The most likely diagnosis is extrinsic allergic alveolitis due to avian precipitins. Budgerigar exposure tends to be low-grade and continuous, hence the presentation is chronic. In contrast, pigeon antigen exposure is heavier and intermittent. Once sensitized, the presentation may be subacute or acute and severe. Raised CRP and ESR, lymphopoenia, raised immunoglobulins and a positive rheumatoid factor are commonly seen. The CXR shows diffuse and poorly defined bilateral alveolar shadowing, changes not typical of miliary TB or sarcoidosis. In any case, these would be unlikely to cause such severe hypoxia. Patients with sarcoidosis are usually quite well. The low KCO effectively excludes vasculitis-related haemorrhage, and there is no eosinophilia. Viral or atypical pneumonia could be the cause, but breathlessness tends to occur late rather than as the presenting symptom. Serology would likely be positive 10 days into the illness. However, PCP would fit the picture well. No information on HIV risk factors is given; thus, although less likely since pigeons are positively mentioned, it is a serious differential not to miss. Forty per cent of pigeon breeders have precipitins, but if positive in this context they would very much strengthen the diagnosis. Bronchoscopy and lavage or biopsy would be hazardous given this degree of hypoxia and would likely necessitate an ICU bed. Hamman–Rich syndrome has historically described the acute variant of idiopathic pulmonary fibrosis, a complex entity that occurs largely in the fifth and sixth decades and relies on histological diagnosis and exclusion of other causes. (N.B. Hamman's sign is the pericardial 'crunch' of pneumonpericardium.)

Case 4.2

1. a
2. e

This is a case of culture-negative endocarditis, probably on a structurally normal native valve. Causes include fastidious organisms such as *Bartonella*, *Coxiella*, HACEK (*Haemophilus*, *Actinobacillus*, *Cardiobacterium*, *Eikenella*, *Kingella*) organisms, and other rare entities such as *Tropheryma whippellii* and *Brucella*. Non-infective causes such as atrial myxomata or non-infective thrombotic endocarditis associated with a connective tissue disorder should also be considered. However, several case series over recent years have highlighted the fairly high prevalence of infection with *Bartonella quintana* among homeless people, apparently transmitted by lice (series in Marseilles and Paris have suggested prevalences between 20 and 50% of current or recent infection). This organism may cause low-grade septicaemia ('trench fever') and endocarditis, as well as peliosis hepatis and bacillary angiomatosis (in immunocompromised patients). In this classical clinical setting, it is deemed the most likely diagnosis. Serology, long-term blood culture (20–40 days) and PCR of affected tissue samples are helpful, as is analysis of captured lice. Synergistic combinations of agents such as erythromycin or tetracycline derivatives in combination with an aminoglycoside are most appropriate. Generally throughout the world, louse-borne infections with agents such as *Borrelia recurrentis* (louse-borne relapsing fever) and *Rickettsia prowazekii* (epidemic typhus) pose a constant latent threat, unmasked by conditions of widespread social upheaval or urban deprivation, as seen recently in Russia and central Africa.

Case 4.3

1. b
2. c

At rest, the principal muscle fuel is free fatty acid, which needs oxygen for metabolism. During strenuous exercise, ATP supply is inadequate and thus glycogen is broken down. If an enzyme is missing, weakness will develop at this point. Adaptation then takes place, through increased blood born glucose and free fatty acid delivery, thus allowing exercise to continue. This 'second-wind phenomenon' is typical of type V glycogen storage disease (McArdle's). Type VII glycogen storage disease is similar to type V but usually presents in childhood. Patients also develop haemolytic anaemia and gout. Type II (acid maltase/Pompe's disease) may present in adults with a painless, progressive proximal myopathy. Diaphragmatic muscle is particularly affected, and a presentation with respiratory failure is not uncommon. Disorders of lipid metabolism may also present only on exercise, as may any of the other causes of myopathic states, although not typically with a 'second wind'.

Case 4.4

1. b
2. b, c, g

Abdominal pain: ?AIP. Polyneuropathy and CNS/SIADH: ?AIP. Abdominal pain is present in 95% of attacks. Autonomic disturbance results in fever, sweating, tachycardia and hypertension. Neuropathy is more commonly motor and usually begins distally, but it may begin in the shoulder girdles. Rapid progression to quadriplegia and respiratory arrest may take place, hence the need to monitor for a decreased vital capacity or hypercarbia. Treatment is with a high carbohydrate intake and intravenous haematin.

Guillain–Barré syndrome may present with back pain severe enough to demand morphine prior to the onset of an obvious peripheral neuropathy (but not abdominal tenderness, as in this case). To confuse matters further, reflexes may be preserved initially (although by the time the neurologist has arrived, things have typically progressed sufficiently to make diagnosis easier–typical!). Nevertheless, patients may need an MRI scan of the thoracic or cervical spine to exclude an acute structural lesion.

Brachial neuritis/amyotrophy presents with pain, often of sudden onset, with a more gradual development of weakness. It may follow an infection or injection and is usually unilateral.

PNH is on the list for 'medical abdominal pains', but nervous system involvement is through CNS haemorrhage or thrombosis.

Vital capacity and blood gases, not peak flow, are the appropriate investigations for respiratory problems due to nervous system disorders.

Case 4.5

1. c
2. a, b

If the patient lives alone, there may be only secondary evidence of nocturnal seizures, such as a wet bed or bruising. The chances of new-onset epilepsy being secondary to a structural lesion are significant at this age. An EEG is therefore of less use, although if it revealed any focal activity and the CT scan was normal, then further imaging with an MRI scan would be mandatory.

Case 4.6

1. c
2. a

Jaundice is provoked by viral hepatitis, fasting, alcohol, menstruation, pregnancy and febrile illness. Hepatitis C infection often leads to chronically mildly raised transaminases, which fluctuate around normal, but the bilirubin is usually not raised. Here, the normal examination, transaminases and haptoglobins make chronic hepatitis or haemolysis unlikely. In Gilbert's syndrome, the hyperbilirubinaemia is unconjugated. A 48-hour fast will generally cause a rise by about 25 μmol/l, while fasting serum bile acids are normal (but raised with most other liver diseases). Nicotinic acid provocation tests have also been used, but the diagnosis is very often one of exclusion. The syndrome occurs in 5–10% of the population and is caused by various different polymorphisms in the promotor region of the UDP glucuronyl transferase gene, reducing the efficiency of bilirubin conjugation in the hepatocytes. *Cryptosporidium* infection can cause sclerosing cholangitis in the context of HIV infection.

Case 4.7

1. c, g
2. a, c

Note the wording would usually say 'renal biopsy – normal'. This is a clue. Think minimal change nephropathy or FSGS. MCN is well known to occur with lymphoma. It usually presents with the nephrotic syndrome. The proteinuria may be highly selective (you may be given urine/plasma ratios of large molecules such as Ig and small molecules such as albumin or transferrin).

Bee stings, grass pollen, poison oak or ivy, and cow's milk have also been implicated in MCN, particularly in atopic individuals. Note that NSAIDs may cause an acute interstitial nephritis, a minimal-change nephrotic syndrome, or a combination of the two.

Other links between malignancy and renal disease include obstruction, chemotherapy hyperuricaemia, chemotherapy toxicity, neoplasia-associated membranous nephropathy, proliferative nephropathy and Henoch–Schönlein purpura nephritis.

Case 4.8

1. d

The patient has a slowly progressive spastic paraplegia and evidence of adrenal insufficiency. The linking diagnosis is an adrenoleukodystrophy. This is a common X-linked recessive disorder that may manifest in the following ways:

*   Familial Addison's disease in males with no neurological involvement, together with a spastic paraparesis in females
*   Cerebral white-matter degeneration, particularly parieto-occipital, in young males with adrenal involvement
*   Progressive spastic paraparesis in adults; 70% have clinical or biochemical evidence of adrenal insufficiency. Low testosterone levels and sphincter disturbance may be present
*   Spastic paraparesis in heterozygote females

The disease is due to a mutation in ABCD1, an ATPase-binding cassette transporter protein. Others in the same family include the gene for cystic fibrosis and the gene for Stargardt disease, a form of macular degeneration. The mutation results in the accumulation of very-long-chain fatty acids, which may be detected in plasma, red blood cells or fibroblasts. DNA analysis can be used to diagnose heterozygotes. Bone marrow transplantation is effective early in the course of the childhood form. Lorenzo's oil has no proven benefit.

Other causes of adrenal insufficiency include:

- TB
- Autoimmune disease
- Metastases
- Lymphoma
- AIDS
- Fungal infection
- CMV
- Amyloidosis
- Haemorrhage in any severe illness
- Haemochromatosis
- Hereditary unresponsiveness to ACTH
- Hypothalamic or pituitary pathology

Note that Addisonian patients may not be hyperkalaemic if they are vomiting and may be hyperglycaemic if the aetiology is autoimmune and associated with diabetes.

Case 4.9

1. d, i, k, r

Appropriate further investigation would include a direct Coombs' test, immunoglobulin levels, bone marrow aspirate and trephine, a blood film and a CT chest. Immune thrombocytopenia may also be seen in around 5% of patients. Fever is unusual in CLL and its presence should trigger a search for infection. The immunoparesis may be multifactorial, often including hypogammaglobulinaemia, neutropenia due to hypersplenism, and more subtle functional defects in cellular immunity. Another cause of fever is transformation, usually to a high-grade non-Hodgkin's lymphoma. This is called Richter's syndrome. Rapid lymph node enlargement and systemic symptoms are common. Note that hypogammaglobulinaemia is a common and treatable cause of late-onset bronchiectasis (remember for clinical cases). This case could also be due to a lymphoma, although this is less likely, particularly in view of the high white cell count. This case would be more taxing were a comprehensive answer to be volunteered rather than chosen from options.

Case 4.10

1. e
2. a

This is a medical emergency. Necrotizing fasciitis can be difficult to recognize in the early stages, but it has a mortality of 20–50%, which appears not to have changed substantially with the advent of potent antibiotics. A painful, swollen, erythematous lesion develops, classically on a limb. The lesion turns purplish-brown before developing haemorrhagic bullae and finally frank necrosis. Lymphangitis and lymphadenopathy are uncommon. Urgent surgical exploration and debridement is the key management step, along with antibiotics and full supportive care. Frozen-section histology and MRI can be useful in the immediate evaluation if available. The lesion is always far more extensive than appears from superficial inspection. Necrotizing fasciitis has been classified according to the offending organism: type 1 (group A *Streptococci*) and type 2 (mixed infection with anaerobes, Gram-negative organisms and enterococci, especially in those debilitated by peripheral vascular problems and diabetes). Necrotizing infections are also prone to develop in the vulva, perineum and scrotum (Fournier's gangrene). A straightforward streptococcal or staphylococcal wound infection is very unlikely to cause toxic shock at this early stage.

Ecthyma gangrenosum is the pathognomonic sign of cutaneous pseudomonas infection, consisting of small haemorrhagic vesicles and progressing to central necrosis and ulceration under a crust. A small minority of patients with pseudomonal bacteraemia suffer this.

Exam 5

Case 5.1

1. c
2. a

Silo filler's lung is a toxic pneumonitis with cough and breathlessness occurring within hours of exposure, sometimes progressing acutely to pulmonary oedema or within weeks to obliterative bronchiolitis. Farmer's lung is characterized by fever, myalgia, cough and breathlessness, four to eight hours post-exposure to mouldy hay. In chronic conditions, there may be no clear history of acute episodes. Crackles and a restrictive infiltrate on CXR are typical. Precipitins may be absent if no exposure has occurred for more than three years. Conversely, 20% of normal farm workers have precipitins. In this case, the breathlessness in the barn and in the evenings fits with both farmer's lung and a dual asthmatic response. However, the absence of lung crepitations, the normal CXR and the (small) response to bronchodilators make asthma due to exposure to barn dust the most likely diagnosis. Moreover, the KCO would be decreased in alveolitis. While the FEV_1/FVC ratio appears restrictive, the RV and TLC are both increased, reflecting air trapping. The FEV_1/FVC ratio viewed on its own can thus be misleading. The poor response to bronchodilators reflects the prominent inflammatory late asthmatic response in action. Steroids are indicated here, and repeat pulmonary function testing after an adequate period of treatment would be valuable. Bronchial provocation testing is done rarely, if ever, and can be dangerous. Occupational asthma patients are sometimes eligible for industrial compensation. Bagassosis and byssinosis are specific types of occupational lung disease caused by exposure to sugar-cane and cotton-derived dusts, respectively.

Case 5.2

1. d

Bacteraemia resulting from infection by invasive serotypes of salmonella is rare but well documented (fewer than 5% of cases). The risk is highest in the elderly. It may result in seeding to bones, joints and aneurysms, but the organism seems to have a particular predilection for atheromatous plaques. Mycotic aneurysms may form some time after the acute gastroenteritis. In persistent infection, or the appropriate clinical context, a search must therefore be made by echocardiography, MRI or angiography for a vascular nidus of infection so surgery can be carried out before fatal rupture occurs. The overall prognosis is poor.

Case 5.3

1. a

Anaemia in the presence of unconjugated hyperbilirubinaemia suggests haemolysis. The good reticulocyte response means there is no aplasia, while the negative Coombs' test means an intrinsic red cell abnormality is likely, with an acute increase in haemolysis. Such a crisis can occur in any patient with shortened red cell survival – i.e. chronic haemolytic state – such as found in sickle cell anaemia, thalassaemia intermedia, hereditary spherocytosis, pyruvate kinase deficiency, etc. While mycoplasma and infectious mononucleosis can cause a similar syndrome, they would cause a positive Coombs' test.

If the reticulocyte count were low, then the picture would be one of pure red cell aplasia. This may be congenital (Diamond–Blackfan syndrome) or acquired. The acquired form is often associated with drugs, thymomas, autoimmune disease and viral infection. The latter is usually due to parvovirus, which has a particular propensity for red cell progenitors. The parvovirus effect is usually noticed only in patients with shortened red cell survival times, i.e. congenital haemolytic anaemia. The other 'crisis' anaemia to remember is the sequestration crisis in sickle cell disease.

Case 5.4

1. d, e, g

Significant right ventricular necrosis occurs in around 20–30% of inferoposterior MIs and may give rise to a venous pressure profile similar to that of pericardial tamponade. In this case, complete heart block has also occurred (the AVN is supplied by the posterior descending artery in 90% of people). Receptors in the inferior myocardium may also mediate hypotension, bradycardia, nausea and vomiting (the Bezold–Jarisch reflex). Diamorphine and, to a lesser extent, frusemide vasodilate and offload particularly the right ventricle. The drop in filling pressure causes the haemodynamic compromise. There is no tachycardic response as the patient is in complete heart block. Mechanical problems such as papillary muscle rupture or VSDs tend to occur later after infarction, once the necrotic myocardium has become more friable (typically around two days after the acute event).

Case 5.5

1. c

The history of episodic overeating, somnolence and hyersexuality is classic for Klein–Levine syndrome. Other behavioural changes may be apparent. Each attack lasts days to, at most, weeks. Most patients have no more than three attacks. Klüver–Bucy syndrome consists of excessive oral exploration of the environment, loss of fear and aggression, and hypersexuality. It results from bilateral amygdala damage.

Case 5.6

1. d
2. b, c (N.B. 'hydrogen breath test' refers to *lactose* hydrogen breath test)

The high stool weight suggests either malabsorption or hypersecretion. The estimated stool osmolality is $2 \times Na + 2 \times K = 300\,mosmol/kg$, which is normal. The calculated value is much higher, suggesting the presence of an unmeasured, osmotically active substance (rather than fluid being secreted). The decreased stool weight on fasting supports this absorptive failure. The commonest causes of osmotic diarrhoea are laxative abuse (e.g. Mg^{2+}) and disaccharidase deficiency. The clues are often in the particular way the history is phrased. It would normally say 'jejunal biopsy was normal', but here it specifically states microscopy. The disaccharidase deficiency is detected by enzymatic assay. The commonest type of deficiency is lactase deficiency. In most populations (of Afro-Asian origin), lactase activity declines after weaning, with symptoms of deficiency developing only if a switch is made to a Western, milk-based diet. Prevalence is as high as 80–90%. Lactase deficiency is less common (estimated prevalence 10–15%) but may develop at any time in people of northern European descent. Any other mucosal disease, e.g. Crohn's, may exacerbate or reveal latent lactase deficiency. Therefore, always consider lactase deficiency in, for example, gastroenteritis or coeliac disease that is slow to respond to appropriate treatment. Breath hydrogen testing after lactose ingestion is a good test: unabsorbed lactose is metabolized by enteric bacteria, releasing hydrogen. The lactose tolerance test (blood glucose profile has minimal rise after lactose ingestion) and the lactose barium meal have high false-positive rates and are no longer used. Rarer disaccharidase deficiencies include sucrase/isomaltase deficiency (sugar- and starch-induced symptoms) and trehalase deficiency (mushroom-induced symptoms).

Case 5.7

1. c
2. b, d

The eosinophilia (implied by the differential cell count) suggests an acute interstitial nephritis and may be associated with eosinophiluria. Common offending drugs include ampicillin, sulphonamides and rifampicin. Recovery usually takes place on stopping the drug and may be hastened by steroids. Fever, flank tenderness, haematuria and sterile pyuria are other common features. Definitive diagnosis requires renal biopsy. A cause of major morbidity after trauma or orthopaedic surgery is fat embolism. Suspect this in a patient with progressive hypoxia or ischaemia/infarction of any organs. The patient typically develops sudden-onset fever, tachycardia and respiratory distress two days after trauma. Fifty per cent have a petechial rash, particularly on the conjunctivae and upper body. Retinal emboli are common. Thrombocytopenia may develop but there is no eosinophilia (in contrast to cholesterol embolism seen in the elderly from complicated atheromata). CNS signs range from confusion to coma, CT showing diffuse oedema. Twenty per cent die and 25% are left with permanent deficits. The other diagnosis to consider is rhabdomyolysis, although this would not explain the eosinophilia and the creatinine would generally be proportionately higher.

Case 5.8

1. d
2. d, i

The clinical picture is of bile duct disease. In an HIV-positive patient, this is most likely to be due to sclerosing cholangitis, which may also be associated with papillitis/papillary stenosis. In this context, infection with CMV or *Cryptosporidium* (and, more rarely, *Microsporidia*, *Isospora* or *Mycobacterium avium intracellulare*) is most likely. These should be sought and treated. Ultrasound, ERCP and biopsy are needed. Acalculous cholecystitis may also be caused by such organisms.

Note that to make a diagnosis of primary sclerosing cholangitis, there must be no gallstones, no previous biliary surgery and sufficient follow-up time to exclude a carcinoma. Patients may have a raised IgM and weakly positive ANA but will be AMA-negative. Presentation may be with cirrhosis and portal hypertension and so should be considered in a cirrhotic patient with cholestatic jaundice. Other common liver disease in advanced HIV infection includes *Mycobacterium avium intracellulare* infection, Kaposi's sarcoma, lymphoma and drug reactions.

Associations of primary sclerosing cholangitis include:

- Inflammatory bowel disease (e.g. an asymptomatic sufferer with a raised ALP)
- Retroperitoneal fibrosis and other idiopathic fibrosing conditions
- Chronic pancreatitis

Other causes of secondary cholangitis include:

- Recurrent bacterial cholangitis
- Injection of caustics into hydatid cysts
- Hepatic arterial cytotoxic infusion

Case 5.9

1. d
2. a, h, i

If patients are ill enough to warrant forced alkaline diuresis, many units will now haemodialyse. Intravenous alkalinization is contraindicated in cases complicated by cerebral or pulmonary oedema. Note that plasma salicylate levels may continue to rise after admission and therefore repeat levels may be necessary if the first level was raised.

Features of salicylate overdose include:

- Tinnitus and deafness
- Blurred vision
- Non-cardiogenic pulmonary oedema
- Cerebral oedema
- Mixed respiratory alkalosis and metabolic acidosis
- Dehydration and acute renal failure
- Low or high glucose
- Low or high sodium
- Deranged clotting
- Convulsions (if severe)
- Myocardial failure

Note: You may be told that the urine Clinitest was positive for glucose. Clinistix specifically detects glucose; Clinitest detects any reducing agent, including salicylates.

Case 5.10

1. e
2. c

Toxic shock syndrome may complicate either carriage of or frank infection by toxin-producing *Staphylococci* or occasionally *Streptococci*. It is associated most infamously with menstruation and colonization of tampons left in situ, but half of cases occur in non-menstruating women or in men. Bacteraemia is rare, and even diligent searches for a nidus of infection may be unproductive. The antibiotics are to eradicate local carriage and as an adjunct to good intensive care. Conventional antistaphylococcal agents such as flucloxacillin are efficacious, while a growing body of evidence suggests that clindamycin may be superior. As pooled immunoglobulin has a high concentration of neutralizing antibodies to the toxin, it may be used in life-threatening cases with some success in addition. Any material – whether it is a dressing, a tampon or a collection of pus – should be removed. Desquamation occurs 10–14 days after the acute illness in survivors. When caused by *Streptococci*, the syndrome is often associated with positive blood cultures. Red cell fragmentation and schistocytes together with anaemia are seen in HUS.

Exam 6

Case 6.1

1. b

0.1% pilocarpine and 2.5% methacholine are too weak to constrict normal pupils but will constrict the Holmes–Adie pupil on account of denervation supersensitivity. If dilating drops had accidentally entered the left eye, then 1% pilocarpine would constrict the right eye but would have no effect on the large pupil. Adrenaline 1:1000 will dilate a postganglionic Horner's pupil but not a normal or a preganglionic Horner's pupil, again because of denervation supersensitivity.

Case 6.2

1. d
2. c
3. b, c

Neurocysticercosis is one of the commonest causes of epilepsy in the developing world. The calcification represents the dead parasite and is not an uncommon incidental finding in endemic areas. It certainly does not preclude a search for other causes, such as alcohol withdrawal here.

The white sclera to the right of the haemorrhage confirms that the blood comes from subconjunctival blood vessels. Battle's sign (bruising behind the ear) is seen several days after a basal skull fracture.

Fresh blood does appear white on CT but would not form discrete dots. Meningiomas arise from the meninges, tend to be larger and more rounded, and are not usually multiple.

Case 6.3

1. e
2. a

The chest film shows an enlarged pulmonary trunk and right ventricle, with peripheral pruning of the pulmonary vasculature. True idiopathic, or primary, pulmonary hypertension is rare, with an incidence of one to two per million. More commonly, it has been associated with appetite suppressant use (especially fenfluramine, phentermine and dexfenfluramine, with an odds ratio of more than 20 after more than three months' use), chronic pulmonary emboli, inhalation of crack cocaine, HIV infection, cirrhosis and a positive family history. After a careful search for a cause, treatment involves anticoagulation to prevent in situ thrombosis, oral vasodilators (often after invasive assessment of their efficacy), intravenous prostacyclin infusion, diuretics with caution, and often ultimately heart–lung transplantation. The prognosis is generally rather poor. The enlarged pulmonary trunk may press on the recurrent laryngeal nerve to cause hoarseness.

Case 6.4

1. a, c
2. d, g

To answer question 2 correctly, you need to consider the differentials for question 1. These were deliberately not included in the list of options for question 1. The two most important differentials are non-convulsive status epilepticus and an organic stupor/abulia. Abulia is a total lack of drive and may occur in certain organic states, e.g. frontal lobe lesions. A normal EEG makes an organic stupor unlikely and excludes non-convulsive status. The positive menace indicates functional connection between retina and cortex, making a psychiatric state more likely.

Note that non-convulsive status is an important treatable cause of 'dementia' or confusion, and it should be considered particularly if the confusion appears to fluctuate or there is a previous history of epilepsy. It is usually due to continuous temporal lobe epileptic activity, and hence there may be no convulsive movements.

Wilson's disease may cause cognitive problems and an extrapyramidal increase in tone. However, in this case the increase in tone is due to a 'voluntary' resistance to movement – often referred to as gegenhalten – commonly seen in confused or demented patients.

Case 6.5

1. b, c, h
2. c

In this case, the whole renin–angiotensin–aldosterone axis is activated. This may be part of the physiological response to underperfusion of all or part of a kidney (proximal stenoses, dehydration, diuretics) or due to paraneoplastic secretion of renin (very rare, from tumours such as haemangiopericytomas or juxtaglomerular apparatus-derived neoplasms; in most cases, renin activity would be extremely high, with more pronounced hypokalaemia, however). In this case, significant aortic coarctation is ruled out by the clinical findings. Beta-blockade reduces renin release from the JGA. The angiogram shows stenosis in the middle of the renal artery, unlike the more proximal or ostial disease seen with atherosclerosis. Most classically, FMD produces multiple distal stenoses, giving a beads-on-a-string appearance. In this case, ACE inhibitors may well be beneficial, or, more definitively, renal angioplasty improves or cures hypertension in 60% of patients with FMD, whereas the effect is more difficult to demonstrate in atherosclerosis. Further functional studies, such as renin response to captopril or MAG3 renograms with captopril, may help to select cases for intervention.

Case 6.6

1. a

The CXR shows a globular cardiac silhouette, and QRS alternans due to swinging of the heart on its pedicle is shown on the ECG. Thus, this question is looking for causes of a pericardial effusion in a patient with AIDS/HIV infection. Of the list presented, TB stands out as the likely cause. Other causes to consider include lymphoma, Kaposi's sarcoma and MAI. TB is the commonest cardiac manifestation of HIV. It may cause an effusion or constrictive pericarditis. Treatment is with antituberculous therapy plus steroids. Surgical removal of the pericardium may be necessary. HIV itself may cause a cardiomyopathy, which occurs late and is usually without symptoms.

Other HIV vignettes:

- HIV-associated thrombocytopoenia: this is common and may revert with antiviral agents. Alternatively, steroids, immunoglobulin, immunoadsoprtion or splenectomy may be necessary
- HIV-associated lupus anticoagulant
- HIV-, varicella zoster virus (VZV)-, herpes simplex virus (HSV)- and CMV-induced myelopathy
- CMV-induced polyradiculopathy
- HIV-associated adrenal insufficiency, e.g. due to TB, CMV, *Cryptococcus* or ketoconazole

Note that common causes of breathlessness include PCP, pulmonary Kaposi's sarcoma, bacterial infections, fungal infections, lymphoma and heart failure.

Patients with CMV anywhere must have their pupils dilated to check for retinitis.

Case 6.7

1. b, f, g

This patient has a lower motor neuron syndrome. MND is most likely, but other disorders must be considered. The most important differentials of a lower motor neuron disorder are multifocal motor neuropathy with conduction block and a cervical radiculopathy, as both are treatable, the former with intravenous immunoglobulin and the latter with surgery. High titres of antiganglioside antibodies are often found in multifocal motor neuropathies with conduction block. If degenerative disease of the cervical spine leads to root compression, then this will result in lower motor neuron signs and is called a cervical radiculopathy. If it leads to cord compression, then upper motor neuron signs result. This is called a cervical myelopathy. If both root and cord compression occur, then the condition is called a mycloradiculopathy. This may mimic forms of MND, with both upper and lower motor neuron signs.

Adult-onset spinal muscular atrophy may be autosomal recessive or autosomal dominant. It is insidious and tends to affect proximal muscles more. Kennedy's syndrome is also called bulbospinal neuronopathy. It is X-linked recessive and presents more slowly, with progressive hand or pelvic girdle weakness. Bulbar involvement may occur, often with grimacing. Gynaecomastia and diabetes may be present. It is due to a CGG repeat expansion in the androgen receptor gene. Myositis almost invariably affects proximal muscles. Inclusion body myositis causes a slowly progressive painless weakness of distal as well as proximal muscles. AIDP (Guillain–Barré syndrome), by definition, reaches its maximum within eight weeks.

Note that a lower motor neuron degeneration may occur some time after radiation therapy. Sensation and sphincter function remain intact. A progressive weakness may also occur many years after polio. This post-polio syndrome may simply reflect a critical lack of reserve neurons to cope with the normal degeneration with age. In young Jews with a motor neuron syndrome, hexosaminidase deficiency should be excluded.

Case 6.8

1. d
2. e
3. c

The area of motor cortex devoted to the foot lies medially. Therefore, bilateral leg weakness with papilloedema is a classic neurological short case of a parasagittal lesion. With such rapid evolution, the most likely diagnosis is a sagittal sinus thrombosis. With a slower evolution, a meningioma is most likely. Tumours can, however, present with sudden onset of symptoms, particularly if there is associated haemorrhage or infarct. A contrast-enhanced CT would be a good first investigation.

Venous thrombosis may present in many different ways and the diagnosis is often missed unless alerted by a well-known syndrome (e.g. idiopathic intracranial hypertension and ear disease – lateral sinus thrombosis; unilateral chemosis, proptosis and ophthalmoplegia – cavernous sinus thrombosis) or the presence of a thrombotic risk factor (e.g. puerperium, sickle cell disease, cyanotic heart disease). Strokes secondary to venous infarction tend to be more haemorrhagic and have greater epileptogenic tendency. In the absence of haemorrhage, anticoagulant therapy may be used.

Case 6.9

1. d

All affected women have affected children. Affected men never have affected children. The best example is Leber's optic neuropathy. Men tend to be affected more severely than women. The other family tree not to be caught out on is that of X-linked dominant inheritance, in which every daughter of an affected male will be affected, unlike the 50% chance with autosomal dominant inheritance, with which it is usually confused.

Case 6.10

1. b

Cortisol is necessary for the distal nephron to excrete a water load. Thus, cortisol deficiency may mask diabetes insipidus. Here, a malignant intracranial deposit is likely causing both ACTH deficiency and diabetes insipidus. Alternatively, lung carcinomas have a predilection for metastasis to the adrenals, which, if extensive, may be the cause of the hypocortisolaemia.

Exam 7

██████████

Case 7.1

1. b

Chest pain in a young man occurring soon after receiving succinylcholine is classically due to succinylcholine myalgia. The pains usually involve the large muscle groups of the chest, back and neck. It is commoner in young patients who mobilize early. As a result of this complication, succinylcholine tends to be used only for cases where the patient will be immobile for at least 24 hours. Credit would be given in a graded scoring system for MI as a diagnosis to exclude.

Case 7.2

1. a

Buruli ulcer occurs in tropical rural areas near rivers, including in Australia. The superficial overhanging ulcer with no constitutional upset, no pain and no lymph-adenopathy is typical. Local ulceration may also result from inoculation with mycobacterium marinum – so-called fish-tank or swimming-pool granuloma. Tropical ulcer is a rather more general description of rapidly progressive ulcers of likely infective origin, which occur predominantly in wet conditions and often contain anaerobic organisms. The purple, overhanging edges of pyoderma gangrenosum are characteristic, while endemic syphilis rarely produces primary skin lesions (gener-ally mucosal, with lymphadenopathy). The raspberry-like primary lesion of yaws does not resemble this. Primary pinta lesions often have satellite lesions and are usu-ally associated with lymphadenopathy.

Case 7.3

1. e
2. c
3. a, b

Drowsy and headache: ?TB. Drowsy and cranial nerve palsies: ?TB. Common predisposing causes for tuberculous meningitis are alcoholism and HIV infection. Other causes of a subacute lymphocytic meningitis are possible, but the time course, CSF analysis and isolated cranial nerve palsy are all highly suggestive of TB. Sarcoidosis usually has mononuclear cells in the CSF. After two weeks of no antibiotics, a bacterial meningitis would have large numbers of polymorphs. Note that the low glucose is a very useful discriminator from viral infection in cases of CSF lymphocytosis.

Clinical features of infection include:

- Deepening coma (may be no meningism)
- Cranial nerve palsies
- Focal neurological deficits
- Raised intracranial pressure
- Spinal cord and nerve root involvement
- Tuberculoma

Mycoplasma-associated neurological syndromes include:

- Cranial neuritis
- Polyneuritis
- Acute myositis
- Aseptic meningitis
- Transverse myelitis
- Encephalomyelitis

The adrenal failure was secondary to adrenal TB.

Case 7.4

1. b
2. b
3. b
4. a
5. b

Giant v waves occur in tricuspid regurgitation because the ventricular contraction is transmitted directly to the large veins. Cannon waves occur when the atria and ventricles contract simultaneously, such as occurs intermittently in complete heart block and other cases of atrioventricular dissociation.

Anion gap = unmeasured anions – unmeasured cations = $(Na + K) - (Cl + HCO_3)$. Causes include renal failure, lactic acidosis, ketoacidosis and exogenous acids (e.g. salicylates).

Many of the features point towards alcohol, but the raised anion gap shifts the diagnosis, at least in the MRCP world, to thiamine deficiency.

Case 7.5

1. e
2. c, e, h, k

The actual patient this is based on had several volumes of notes and was due to have long-acting epidural local anaesthetic injections. Her abdominal X-ray showed calcification and her pain improved greatly with enzyme supplements.

The pain of chronic pancreatitis is very variable. It may be chronic or remitting. Food may exacerbate the pain and result in anorexia. Some patients have signs of malabsorption and some have only steatorrhoea with no pain. Investigations should look at structure (e.g. CT and ERCP) and function (both endocrine and exocrine) as well as seeking complications such as deficiency of fat-soluble vitamins. The treatment for pain and steatorrhoea is the same: abstain from alcohol and supplement enzymes. If patients are given sufficient doses of enzyme supplementation, then 75% will be rendered pain-free. Note that complications of chronic pancreatitis such as osteomalacia may themselves cause bone pain.

Case 7.6

1. d

Even if you have never heard of a hepatic wedge pressure, you can work out that if it is normal in the face of portal hypertension (splenomegaly and varices), then the underlying disease must be presinusoidal. The septic episode after surgery close to the biliary tree gives a strong clue. The open cholecystectomy might date the operation to the days when blood was not screened for hepatitis C carriage. Hepatitis C cirrhotics may have no clinical signs and may have normal liver function tests. However, the cirrhosis is intrahepatic, involving both pre- and post-sinusoidal liver; thus, the wedge pressure would be raised. Likewise with chronic non-alcoholic steatohepatitis (NASH) (suspected widely to be the most common cause of 'cryptogenic' cirrhosis), alcohol-related cirrhosis and PBC (although the signs of chronic liver disease are much more prominent in the latter two). That the hypertension is presinusoidal means that liver function will be more preserved and thus shunting operations less likely to be complicated by the development of encephalopathy. Note that in post-sinusoidal hypertension due to hepatic vein thrombosis (Budd–Chiari syndrome – think ?PNH), blood is diverted through the caudate lobe, which drains more directly into the IVC. Splenic vein thrombosis usually occurs in the context of pancreatitis or gastric surgery, but it can be spontaneous and should be considered here. It may cause isolated gastric or oesophageal varices with normal livers.

Case 7.7

1. d
2. d
3. a, e
4. f

The brain scan is an axial T2-weighted MRI, showing a space-occupying lesion with surrounding oedema and mass effect. Note that the CSF is white, as it is a T2-weighted image. The fluid from the oedema is therefore also white. In a patient with AIDS, a space-occupying lesion is treated as being due to toxoplasmosis. If there is no response to anti-tuberculous therapy in a week, then consideration is given to biopsy. Toxoplasma serology will not distinguish current from past infection. If the imaging is normal, then a lumbar puncture should be undertaken. Cryptococcal meningitis can be very insidious and may present with only headache and no neck stiffness or with focal signs. Cocci are seen with CSF India ink stain in 70%, whereas Cryptococcal antigen is detected in blood or CSF in nearly 100%. TB, HSV, CMV, syphilis, bacteria and malignancy are alternative diagnoses to consider in the case of a normal CT. Progressive multifocal leukoencephalopathy may present with a rapid progression of personality deterioration, seizures and focal deficits, although it can also present rather slowly and appear as a mass lesion initially on CT without any obvious demyelination. It is due to the JC virus, which causes massive demyelination. Note that Kaposi's sarcomas are extremely rare in intravenous drug-users, since the herpes virus associated with Kaposi's sarcomas is sexually transmissible and appears to be of low prevalence in this population, but it is much more common in gay men and in African men and women.

Case 7.8

1. b, c, f

The two principal differential diagnoses are MND and a cervical myelopathy. Given the previous STD history and the fact that it is treatable, spinal syphilis also enters the differential here. In this case, there is a mix of upper motor neuron signs and lower motor neuron signs in the absence of sensory signs, suggesting MND. In making the diagnosis of MND, one looks for a mix of upper and lower motor neuron signs in the same limb, and therefore the brisk reflex of a wasted muscle is very significant and indeed the 'normal' upper limb reflexes in the wasted muscles in this case may well reflect a degree of hyperreflexia. Patients may have sensory symptoms but not sensory signs. The diagnosis becomes apparent with follow-up, but it may mimic several other conditions at presentation (*vide infra*). A cervical myelopathy enters the differential. It is unlikely given the lack of pain or sensory signs, but it is not a diagnosis you would want to miss. EMG would be useful in this particular case, as detection of denervation over many segments would be more in keeping with MND. Syphilitic arachnoiditis may cause upper-limb amyotrophy and lower-limb long tract signs. A pure lower motor neuron syphilitic amyotrophy may also occur.

Presentations of MND to be wary of include (common misdiagnosis given in inverted commas):

- The weak or stiff hand
- Foot drop ('peroneal nerve palsy')
- Proximal weakness ('muscular dystrophy')
- Weak neck, thoracic or trunk muscles
- Single spastic limb or ipsilateral limbs ('hemiplegia')

Case 7.9

1. b

Whipple's triad (fasting hypoglycaemia, hypoglycaemic symptoms, and relief with glucose) is the classical triad of insulinomas. Symptoms may be autonomic (sweating, palpitation, irritability) or neuroglycopoenic (e.g. confusion, slurred speech, amnesia, coma, convulsions) and may be associated with weight gain due to the learned ability to abolish symptoms with food. Diagnosis, as is generally true in endocrinology, must first be biochemical, with the demonstration of adequate fasting hypoglycaemia (<2.2 mmol/l) with concomitant hyperinsulinaemia and appropriately elevated C peptide or pro-insulin (this gives extra information, as an elevated pro-insulin/insulin ratio is characteristic of insulinomas). Even if endogenous hyperinsulinaemia is proven, it is imperative to screen simultaneous specimens of urine and blood for sulphonylureas and, if possible, meglitinides, especially if the patient has access to these agents. Otherwise, a 72-hour fast, if conducted well, approaches 100% sensitivity for diagnosis. Glucagon testing and urine/blood ketone testing are useful confirmation of adequate fasting.

Case 7.10

1. c

The syndrome consists of multiple vocal and motor tics that change with time, often with coprolalia (grunts becoming obscenities), echolalia, copropraxia (involuntary obscene gesturing), palilalia and echopraxia. Many patients have obsessive-compulsive features. Note that the syndrome should really be called Gilles de la Tourette syndrome, as this was the surname of the describer (his first name was George, not Gilles).

Exam 8

Case 8.1

1. a, i

Malignant hyperpyrexia and tetany are possible answers, but they are not the best-fit diagnoses from the list.

There are four syndromes that closely resemble one another: neuroleptic malignant syndrome, malignant hyperpyrexia, serotonin syndrome and an ecstasy syndrome. Malignant hyperpyrexia is an autosomal dominant trait that needs to be considered in all unexplained cases of tachycardia, sweating, hyperventilation and cyanosis. It may present with rigidity after suxamethonium administration or with failure of the masseters to relax pre-intubation. The latter features are equivalent to the neuroleptic malignant syndrome. It may develop with muscle relaxants, inhalational and local anaesthetics, plus a range of other drugs. The likely mechanism is failure to take up calcium from the myoplasm, resulting in continual muscle contraction. Treatment is active cooling, dantrolene and ventilation. Severe metabolic acidosis is common and should be treated with sodium bicarbonate. Rhabdomyolysis may result.

The neuroleptic malignant syndrome is similar, although it develops more insidiously and pyrexia may be absent initially. It is an idiosyncratic reaction to therapeutic doses of agents affecting CNS dopaminergic transmission such as phenothiazines and butyrophenones. The predisposition is not genetically inherited. The treatment is the same as for malignant hyperpyrexia, although in view of the central origin of the increased tone neuromuscular junction paralysis may be effective.

The serotonin syndrome was recognized only in 1991. Combinations of drugs acting on serotonin receptors, typically fluoxetine and an MAOI, result in hyperstimulation of central $5HT_{1a}$ receptors, leading to rigidity, tremor, hyperthermia, autonomic disturbance, myoclonus, DIC and rhabdomyolysis. Treatment is with benzodiazepines and beta-blockers.

Ecstasy acts on both dopaminergic and serotonergic neurons. It may cause an unpredictable and rapid rigidity, hyperthermia, trismus and tachycardia, leading on to rhabdomyolysis, DIC and renal failure.

Case 8.2

1. d
2. d

The normal platelet count effectively excludes DIC. In DIC, the APTT and PT are markedly prolonged, with FDPs of typically 0.5–1.5 g/l. In contrast, the very low fibrinogen, high FDP level but only minimally prolonged APTT and PT suggest primary fibrinolysis (in this situation, the D dimer level is usually normal). The distinction is not always this clear-cut. A short euglobin clot lysis time is a good screen for fibrinolytic activation. Prostatic and pelvic tissues are rich in tissue plasminogen activator (tPA), which may be released during surgery or from metastatic tumours. tPA clearance is reduced in liver cirrhosis. Treatment is with plasma replacement and anti-fibrinolytic agents. DDAVP is used to boost factor VIII levels in von Willebrand's disease and mild haemophilia A, but it can increase levels of fibrinolysis. Inappropriate use of fibrinolytic inhibitors in DIC may result in catastrophic widespread thrombosis.

Causes of primary fibrinolysis include:

- Pelvic and prostate surgery
- Dental extractions
- Liver transplantation
- Cardiopulmonary bypass
- tPA, streptokinase, urokinase
- Acute promyelocytic leukaemia
- Congenital deficiency of plasminogen activator inhibitor (PAI)

Case 8.3

1. a

Causes of prolonged bleeding time include:

- Low number of platelets
- Abnormal platelet function:
  - Abnormal adhesion, e.g. Von Willebrand's disease, Bernard–Soulier syndrome
  - Abnormal aggregation, e.g. Glanzmann's thrombasthenia, afibrinogenaemia, drugs (ticlopidine, anti-glycoprotein IIb/IIIa agents such as abciximab), dysproteinaemia
  - Abnormal platelet release, e.g. reduced cyclo-oxygenase activity (aspirin, NSAIDs, congenital), storage pool diseases, uraemia, platelet coating (e.g. penicillins), mixed disorders
- Connective tissue disorders
- Factor V deficiency
- Liver failure

This lady has had a painful tooth and has probably taken analgesics as well as penicillin to cover the dental procedure. Therefore, the most likely diagnosis is drug-induced platelet dysfunction. Connective tissue disorders are excluded by examination. Bernard–Soulier syndrome and the grey platelet syndrome are associated with large platelets. Factor V deficiency also causes a marked prolongation of PT and APTT. Acquired platelet granule depletion (storage pool disease) is associated with autoimmune disease. However, storage pool disease and Glanzmann's thrombasthenia (glycoprotein IIb/IIIa deficiency) have abnormal aggregation to ADP, in contrast to aspirin. Fibrinogen disorders would produce a prolonged thrombin time. Type 2 von Willebrand's disease features normal levels of antigen but impaired function (and therefore impaired ristocetin-induced platelet aggregation). After aspirin ingestion, platelet aggregation in response to collagen is impaired at low doses.

Note: a slide of a fair child (albino) with recurrent nose bleeds: ?Hermansky–Pudlak syndrome.

Note: a slide of a fair child (albino) with recurrent infections: ?Chediak–Higashi syndrome.

Case 8.4

1. c

The autonomic nerve fibres, pain and temperature sensation travel in small peripheral nerve fibres and, if affected selectively, do not lead to dropped reflexes. Autonomic features may be a prominent feature in the more common neuropathies, such as:

- AIP
- Diabetes mellitus
- Amyloidosis
- Alcohol
- Nutritional deficits
- Chronic inflammatory demyelinating polyneuropathy
- Guillain–Barré syndrome

Case 8.5

1. e
2. e

Both cholecystitis and hepatitis cause a leukocytosis, fever, right upper quadrant pain, nausea and jaundice. The hepatomegaly and raised liver enzymes strongly suggest hepatitis as the cause. The clues towards an alcoholic aetiology include the rib fractures, AST to ALT ratio of greater than two, and the disproportionately raised GGT. Many cases show cholestasis. Liver biopsy provides the definitive diagnosis where this is not clear from clinical and biochemical grounds as well as simple imaging. The use of corticosteroids in alcoholic hepatitis, while somewhat controversial, is often advocated when the discriminant function* is greater than 32, and/or in the presence of hepatic encephalopathy, and when infection, gastrointestinal bleeding and renal failure have been excluded.

Case 8.6

1. b, f
2. a, b

The two commonest causes of fever in advanced disease are MAC and lymphoma. MAC is of low virulence and usually only becomes a problem with severe immunocompromise, with CD4 counts below 50/mm³. However, in the era of Highly Active Antiretroviral Therapy, there are increasing numbers of patients recognized who, within a few months of starting therapy, suffer massive lymph node swelling as a reaction to existing *Mycobacterium avium intracellulare*, which may resemble lymphoma both clinically and radiologically. It may be detected with special blood culture techniques or with an acid-fast stain of lymph node, liver or bone marrow. ALP is often raised significantly, while the other liver function tests may be normal. MAC may be present in the faeces without disseminated infection. Modern regimens often include MAC prophylactic agents such as clarithromycin. CT abdomen is necessary to look for lymphoma. Sometimes the cause of the fever is not found and it is ascribed to HIV itself. Generalized wasting (more than 10% weight loss, with intermittent or constant fever and chronic fatigue or diarrhoea for more than 30 days without a cause apparent apart from HIV infection) is the initial AIDS-defining illness in the USA in 9% of patients and is currently the leading initial clinical manifestation of AIDS. It is a diagnosis of exclusion. The lack of focal signs and drug prophylaxis make pneumocystis and toxoplasmosis (co-trimoxazole) and cryptococcosis (fluconazole) less likely.

Note: leg pain and weakness in HIV: ?AZT myopathy.

Note: shortness of breath/desaturation on exercise but clear chest: ?PCP.

Note: diarrhoea with normal stool culture: ?cryptosporidiosis (need acid-fast stain). Other causes of diarrhoea are *Isospora belli*, microsporidia, MAC, CMV colitis, autonomic neuropathy, HIV gastropathy and drug side effects.

Case 8.7

1. e
2. b

---

* Most commonly 4.6 × (prolongation of prothrombin time) + [bilirubin]/17.

Whenever chloride and bicarbonate values are given, calculate the anion gap. Here, there is a hyperkalaemic normal anion gap acidosis. This is termed type IV RTA. It may be due to interference with aldosterone action, e.g. spironolactone, aldosterone resistance (pseudohypoaldosteronism) or decreased capacity of the adrenals to synthesize aldosterone. Most commonly, however, it is due to hyporeninaemia. This may occur in many chronic renal diseases, particular those damaging the interstitium, or it may be due to drugs such as beta-blockers or those interfering with prostaglandin synthesis. Despite low levels of secreted acid, low ammonia levels in the urine decrease buffering capacity, and so the urine pH can fall below 5.5. With gastrointestinal bicarbonate loss, renal compensation gives rise to a negative urine anion gap.

Thus, the classic case for type 4 RTA is a diabetic lady on a NSAID. As renal disease progresses, and the GFR drops below 50% normal, other anions such as phosphate and sulphate are retained, so a raised anion gap develops despite low levels of aldosterone action. Treatment may involve fludrocortisone, a high salt/low sodium diet, a loop diuretic, and cessation of contributing drugs such as spironolactone and NSAIDs.

Causes of RTA type IV include:

- Decreased renin production
- Chronic tubulointerstitial nephritis
- Diabetes mellitus
- NSAIDs
- ACE inhibitors
- Beta-blockers
- Adrenal disease
- Addison's disease
- Inborn errors of steroid metabolism
- Spironolactone
- Pseudohypoaldosteronism

Case 8.8

1. a
2. a

The disc margin is blurred. Exudates radiate out from the disc. There are also two haemorrhages superiorly. The fundal appearances of optic neuritis and papilloedema are very similar. The conditions are distinguished by the fact that papilloedema is usually bilateral while optic neuritis is usually unilateral. Also, optic neuritis is often painful and associated with marked visual loss. Here, the history is classical for the transient visual obscurations of idiopathic intracranial hypertension. Visual impairment usually begins with an enlargement of the blind spot, followed by peripheral field constriction, acuity decline occurring late. However, severe visual loss may still occur, sometimes rapidly and unpredictably, hence the name idiopathic intracranial hypertension (IIH) rather than benign intracranial hypertension (BIH).

The sixth nerve palsy is a false localizing sign. With the absence of any other neurological signs, the likelihood of a space-occupying lesion is small. Therefore, while one can only say this patient has raised intracranial pressure, the most likely diagnosis is IIH. The diagnosis is confirmed by a normal CT, with a raised opening pressure at lumbar puncture and normal CSF analysis. Treatment is to remove any underlying cause and drain CSF through repeated lumbar punctures. If these measures fail, some use prednisolone, acetazolamide or frusemide. Occasionally, the coperitoneal shunting or optic nerve sheath fenestration is necessary to preserve vision. The majority of patients are young, overweight females with menstrual irregularities. Losing weight would probably be effective but is seldom achieved quickly enough. Visual obscuration is a feature of papilloedema, not specifically of BIH.

Other causes of raised intracranial pressure include:

- Vitamin A toxicity (especially isotretinoin)
- Vitamin A deficiency
- Tetracycline overdose
- Lead poisoning
- Corticosteroid withdrawal
- Venous sinus thrombosis
- Oestrogens
- Phenothiazines
- Hypo/hyperadrenalism
- Hypothyroidism
- Hypoparathyroidism
- Guillain–Barré syndrome
- Chronic meningitis

Note that chronic meningitis may not show up on a scan; therefore, CSF analysis is needed to exclude a chronic meningitis such as sarcoidosis, tuberculosis or malignancy. Many recommend imaging to exclude sinus thrombosis in patients with IIH, particularly if there is any risk factor. Note that an average of 500 ml of CSF is produced each day. Lumbar puncture headaches are therefore due to the amount of CSF that subsequently leaks out through the needle track (i.e. needle gauge) rather than the amount of CSF removed.

Case 8.9

1. a, c
2. b, e

The history of recurrent weakness the night after heavy exercise in the absence of sensory loss suggests a periodic paralysis. Myasthenia gravis must always be considered in any patient with variable, intermittent or fatiguable weakness and is the principal differential from this list. A metabolic myopathy is also possible, although the timing and lack of muscle breakdown (normal CK, no myoglobinuria) make this less likely. AIP is another possibility, although it is not listed here. If his exercise exacerbated some vertebral instability, then a recurrent cervical myelopathy could be a possibility, although again the timing, lack of pain, sensory loss and history of trauma makes this very unlikely. Guillain–Barré syndrome (acute inflammatory demyelinating polyneuropathy is the same condition) is monophasic. The related chronic inflammatory demyelinating polyneuropathy may be relapsing but with a time course of weeks or months. The periodic paralyses typically commence in adolescence, with weakness developing overnight after heavy exercise, particularly if followed by a carbohydrate load. Attacks diminish in severity with age. Hypokalaemic, hyperkalaemic and, rarely, normokalaemic syndromes are recognized. The hypokalaemic variety is associated with thyrotoxicosis. In myasthenia, a clinically weak muscle needs to be in evidence for a Tensilon test to be carried out. An anti-acetylcholine receptor antibody titre is an easier investigation than an EMG, although there is a false-negative rate with antibody testing approaching 50% in isolated ocular myasthenia. Anti-MUSK (muscle-specific tyrosine kinase) antibodies are detectable in a percentage of anti-acetylcholine receptor-negative patients.

Case 8.10

1. a, d

Fabry's disease is due to lysosomal accumulation of alpha-galactosyl-lactosyl-ceramide. It is X-linked recessive. Hemizygote females may be asymptomatic or may show any of the disease characteristics, usually with less severity. Features include burning peripheral pain and paraesthesiae provoked by temperature change and exercise, progressive renal impairment, stroke and MI. Raynaud's phenomenon, abdominal and musculoskeletal pains, avascular necrosis and lung infiltration may also occur. The characteristic rash is angiokeratoma corporis diffusum. A corneal dystrophy with characteristic slit-lamp appearance is seen (verticillata – also seen with amiodarone, chloroquine and indomethacin).

Exam 9

Case 9.1

1. b

This presentation in a young, fit, Western European man fits best with an acute infective mesenteric adenitis/ileitis. Patients with viral infections may develop generalized lymphadenitis and abdominal pain, with enlarged mesenteric nodes found at laparotomy. EBV infection can present as an acute abdomen due to mesenteric adenitis alone, but such abdominal signs together with the mesenteric hyperaemia strongly suggest a local cause. *Campylobacter* infection gives rise to an inflamed, oedematous ileum, but it may spread to the colon and mimic ulcerative colitis and cause enlarged mesenteric nodes. Likewise, *Salmonella* species cause an enteritis. Note that patients with mesenteric adenitis or ileitis from *Yersinia* often do not have any diarrhoea at all. *Y. pseudotuberculosis* usually presents acutely or subacutely with mesenteric adenitis in contrast to *Y. enterocolitica*, which presents thus in about 20%, the more typical syndrome being that of an enteritis. Diagnosis may be made by acute and convalescent *Yersinia* serology, and fresh wet stool smear and culture. Uncomplicated *Yersinia* enterocolitis or pseudoappendicitis needs no treatment. If necessary, a quinolone or tetracycline is appropriate pending sensitivities.

Case 9.2

1. b
2. a

The visual fields show a central scotoma involving the macula in the left eye and a small loss of the upper outer visual quadrant in the right eye. Often, the scotoma is believed to be more acute than it is because of the sudden accidental discovery. The optic atrophy suggests a more chronic process. In external compression of the optic nerve, the papillomacular bundle is particularly sensitive, resulting initially in a scotoma. The other vulnerable fibres are those crossing over in the anterior chiasm. Thus, the early upper temporal field deficit in the opposite eye is very suggestive of extrinsic optic nerve/anterior chiasmal compression, e.g. from a tuberculum sella meningioma. If intrinsic compression occurs, think optic nerve glioma in neurofibromatosis.

Case 9.3

1. a
2. f

The signs initially suggest a hereditary degenerative disorder, but the myopathy does not fit. The clues are the glue-sniffer's rash from the crisp packet placement and the drunk-like appearance.

Complications of volatile substance abuse include:

- Drunk-like appearance
- Convulsions
- Cerebellar signs
- Neuropathy
- Optic atrophy
- Altered mental state
- Abdominal pain
- Haematemesis
- Aplastic anaemia
- Rhabdomyolysis
- Hypokalaemia
- Hypophosphataemia
- Acute hepatic and renal damage
- Renal tubular acidosis

Case 9.4

1. c
2. d

The signs are bilateral and all lower motor neuron. Saddle anaesthesia with sphincter disturbance suggests sacral roots or cauda equina pathology. Conus lesions usually have mixed upper and lower motor neuron signs, e.g. an extensor plantar. Bilateral sacral plexus lesions large enough to cause this deficit are rare. Some pain would be expected with a central disc prolapse. Dysraphism refers to disorders associated with failure of fusion of the midline structure from the neural tube. Some of the associated cysts and tumours are implicated in a late progressive cauda equina syndrome on account of cord tethering. Other intramedullary tumours include ependymomas, meningiomas and neurofibromas, although extradural metastases and lymphomas are overall more common.

Case 9.5

1. b, c, f
2. c
3. b

The VDRL may be negative during early infection, and it becomes negative or falls to a low titre with successful treatment. It is therefore a useful marker of disease activity. False-positive responses are usually of low titre (1/8 or less). TPHA and FTA-Abs are specific anti-treponemal tests, become positive earlier than VDRL, and usually remain positive. False-positives are rare. However, they do not discriminate between venereal syphilis and endemic syphilis, yaws or pinta. VDRL and IgG FTA-Abs transfer passively across the placenta, but TPHA and IgM FTA-Abs do not. HIV infection may delay syphilis seroconversion. Secondary syphilis occurs within a few months at the latest of the primary stage. Therefore, if this were secondary syphilis she must have been reinfected. Chancroid, caused by *Haemophilus ducreyi*, causes painful ulceration, with tender, suppurating local lymphadenopathy, unlike the painless chancre and lymphadenopathy of syphilis.

HIV infection is a cause of false-positive VDRL. ELISA has a sensitivity of over 99%, but specificity is as low as 13%, so a positive test is followed by a confirmatory test such as Western blot for p24, gp41 and gp120/160. Western blotting is less useful for following up a negative test, in which case repeat testing in three months is recommended. Alternatively, p24 capture assay will pick up 50% of those yet to seroconvert, while HIV nucleic acid detection has the highest sensitivity at this stage. ELISA is useful from 18 months onwards in cases of vertical transmission due to transplacental antibody passage.

Case 9.6

1. b
2. d

Pathologically, IgA nephropathy and HSP form part of a clinical spectrum. One or more of polyarthritis, abdominal symptoms (pain, bleeding, obstruction from haematomas or intussusception) and skin lesions (limb and buttock urticaria/ purpura/necrosis) following a recent infection suggest the diagnosis of HSP, hence this is deemed the most accurate diagnosis here. Nephritic syndrome, nephrotic syndrome or macroscopic haematuria may be apparent. IgA and C3 deposition is seen in the skin lesions or glomeruli (but skin biopsy is substantially less hazardous than renal biopsy). Serum IgA is raised in 50%. IgA nephropathy usually occurs 12–24 hours after an infection involving an IgA-protected mucosal surface (pharynx, breast, genital tract, gut, bronchus). In contrast, post-streptococcal glomerulonephritis occurs 10–14 days after an infection. Of note, there is a condition of persistent microscopic haematuria defined by the finding of a thin membrane seen only on electron microscopy. It is benign and familial and is called thin-membrane nephropathy. Episodes of macroscopic haematuria may occur, and it therefore enters the differential of IgA disease and Alport's syndrome.

Case 9.7

1. a

Both the plasma and urine osmolalities are low. This can only be from drinking too much. Almost invariably this is psychogenic in origin, although sarcoidosis is a rare organic cause. There is some evidence that a subset of people have an abnormal osmotic thirst threshold but normal ADH secretion and renal function. Long-term polydipsia can impair the renal capacity to concentrate urine.

Lithium may cause nephrogenic diabetes insipidus, hypercalcaemia, renal tubular acidosis and hypothyroidism (15% of treated patients).

Case 9.8

1. c
2. a

This lady has features of CREST (calcinosis, Raynaud's, oesophageal dysmotility, sclerodactyly and telangiectasia) syndrome, most commonly found in limited cutaneous scleroderma. This variant of systemic sclerosis is characterized by distal and acral skin involvement only, less visceral disease, and a better prognosis than diffuse cutaneous scleroderma. In less than 10% of patients after 10 years of disease, isolated pulmonary hypertension develops, with a poor prognosis. In this case, the ECG shows the right ventricular strain pattern characteristic of this condition. More common is pulmonary fibrosis with mild secondary pulmonary hypertension. Primary biliary cirrhosis is a further association. In diffuse cutaneous scleroderma, isolated pulmonary hypertension is much rarer, although fibrosis is slightly more common. Oesophageal stasis predisposes to aspiration. Scleroderma may also be complicated by pneumothoraces, haemorrhage and scar carcinomas. Note that patients with diffuse cutaneous scleroderma may present acutely with diffuse itchy skin swelling. If headaches or visual disturbance are present, then consider hypertensive renal crisis urgently. Patients should be taking an ACE inhibitor. Sixty to eighty per cent of patients with limited disease have positive anticentromere antibodies.

Case 9.9

1. c, d
2. c
3. b, e

Orthopnoea is seen most commonly in cardiogenic pulmonary oedema. It is also characteristic of bilateral diaphragmatic weakness and is rarely a feature of obstructive airway disease. Perfusion–diffusion mismatching in the hyperdynamic pulmonary circulation of hepatic cirrhosis can lead to deoxygenation on standing, while lack of abdominal musculature denies the diaphragm its usual splinting and results in platypnoea (breathlessness on standing). Pleuritic pain in SLE typically lasts days and is often accompanied by pericarditis. The shrinking lung syndrome refers to a restrictive ventilatory defect with dyspnoea and orthopnoea due to an elevated diaphragm, which is seen to move poorly on fluoroscopic screening. The cause is understood incompletely, but myopathy or myositis of the diaphragm and/or phrenic nerve dysfunction are implicated most often, with atelectasis developing secondarily. Other explanations put forward are multiple small vasculitis-related infarcts and primary atelectasis.

Respiratory complications of SLE include:

- Pleurisy/effusions
- Bronchiolitis obliterans
- Diffuse interstitial pneumonitis
- Diaphragmatic myopathy
- Basal atelectasis
- Pulmonary vasculitis and haemorrhage
- Increased risk of infection
- Pulmonary hypertension

Case 9.10

1. d
2. a

Cataplexy is the sudden loss of muscle tone brought on by emotion. Patients often develop phlegmatic personalities for their own protection. It is part of the tetrad of narcolepsy (with sleep attacks, sleep paralysis, and hypnogogic or hypnopompic hallucinations) and is due to the atonia of REM sleep intruding into waking life.

It usually lasts only seconds, but it may last hours (status cataplecticus). Cataplexy may, on occasion, begin before the somnolence. It enters the differential of drop attacks, although the occurrence with emotion and preservation of consciousness make the diagnosis easy. A possibly related condition is incontinence during laughter in children (giggle micturition); certainly, children may on occasion lose tone if tickled enough. In the absence of cataplexy, narcolepsy is diagnosed by the sleep latency test. An autosomal dominant form of narcolepsy exists in Doberman pinschers and Labradors. The gene is the hypocretin receptor. Amphetamines or modafinil treat the sleepiness, while tricyclics treat the cataplexy.

Exam 10

████████

Case 10.1

1. a
2. e

Chylous fluid is classically described as milky and opalescent, due to the presence of fat globules. It may be confused with an empyema (when the cells are spun down, a clear supernatant remains) or pseudochyle. The latter is due to the high lipid (usually cholesterol) levels of some chronic effusions, most typically tuberculous effusions. The commonest causes of chylothorax are trauma (including surgery) and malignancy. The malignancy is usually lymphoma. Less commonly, metastatic deposits, often from stomach cancer, are the cause. Investigation should include a thoracic CT scan and if, necessary, a lymphangiogram. Prolonged chest drainage can result in malnutrition and immunodeficiency.

Other causes of chylothorax include:

- Congenital absence of thoracic duct
- Filariasis
- Tuberculous mediastinal lymphadenitis
- Yellow nail syndrome
- Left subclavian vein thrombosis
- Lymphangioleiomyomatosis
- Miscellaneous compression of the thoracic duct (thoracic aortic aneurysms, large goitre, etc.)

Case 10.2

1. c
2. b

Langerhan's cell histiocytosis is now the preferred term for the spectrum of disease previously covered by terms such as Letterer–Siwe disease, Hand–Schuller–Christian disease and histiocytosis X. It may be a single- or multisystem disorder. It can present at any age and is underdiagnosed. Resolution of lesions, particularly in single-system disease, is often spontaneous. Diagnosis is histological, most usually from skin or bone biopsy. The commonest presentation of pulmonary disease is with non-productive cough and dyspnoea, and one-third of such patients have constitutional symptoms such as weight loss and fever. Five to fifteen per cent of patients with pulmonary disease have symptoms from other organ systems. CXR usually shows bilateral mid- and upper-zone reticulonodular infiltrates in early disease, with late disease sometimes closely resembling emphysema with cystic changes. High-resolution CT of the chest can provide sufficient diagnostic information in the correct clinical context to avoid lavage and biopsy.

Clinical features include:

- Failure to thrive
- Painful bone swelling (X-ray: well-defined osteolytic lesion)
- Rash (often mistaken for cradle cap or seborrhoeic eczema)
- Lymphadenopathy
- Hepatomegaly
- Splenomegaly
- Interstitial lung disease
- Otitis externa
- CNS (often pituitary/hypothalamic or cerebellar)
- Any part of gastrointestinal tract

Case 10.3

1. d
2. g
3. a

Alport's syndrome often presents with microscopic haematuria, becoming macroscopic after infection or exercise. Urinary frequency or a nephrotic state may precede progressive renal failure. It is usually X-linked dominant. It is associated with lenticonus (appears as cataract at a distance, disappearing as the ophthalmoscope approaches the eye), macular abnormalities, leiomyomatosis, macrothrombocytopoenia and sensorineural deafness. The deafness may be slight or present only in other family members with no renal problems. The molecular defect is a mutation in a collagen subunit of the basement membrane. Rarely, alloimmunization to the normal subunit on a transplanted kidney develops, with a resultant antiglomerular basement membrane crescentic glomerulonephritis.

IgA nephropathy, the commonest primary glomerular cause of end-stage renal disease, usually presents with recurrent macroscopic haematuria within 24 hours of an upper respiratory tract infection (or infection involving other IgA-protected mucosal surfaces). Diagnosis is confirmed by renal biopsy, not by serology. Although previously considered relatively benign, prognosis is variable, with 15–50% progressing to end-stage renal disease (usually slowly, but occasionally rapidly).

(Pendred's syndrome is a red herring, consisting of the association of sensorineural deafness and goitre, sometimes with hypothyroidism, due to mutation of the pendrin gene.)

Case 10.4

1. a
2. a, g

The diagnosis requires five of the following features (four if there are proven coronary aneurysms):

- Fever of unknown origin for more than five days
- Polymorphous rash
- Cervical lymphadenopathy
- Bilateral conjunctival congestion
- Dry, red or fissured lips/erythematous buccal cavity
- Peripheral oedema/redness/desquamation

Treatment is with aspirin (a situation where the fear of Reye's syndrome is superseded) and high-dose gammaglobulin to prevent cardiac complications (coronary aneurysms, myocarditis, pericarditis, cardiac failure). Note that in practice this condition is often difficult to sort out from the other viral exanthems, but if there is any clinical suspicion echocardiography should be performed at the earliest opportunity.

Case 10.5

1. b, f
2. a

The malabsorption picture together with a history of chronic infections at mucosal surfaces and the radiological appearance suggest a diagnosis of nodular lymphoid hyperplasia. Nodular lymphoid hyperplasia is seen with hypogammaglobulinaemia. Only IgA may be low. An absence of plasma cells is seen on biopsy. Villi are usually normal, but subtotal villous atrophy may develop. IgA deficiency occurs with a frequency of one in 600 in European populations. It may occur secondary to phenytoin or penicillamine use and in protein-losing enteropathies. It is associated with several gastrointestinal disorders, including:

- Infection, e.g. giardia, bacterial overgrowth
- Pernicious anaemia

- Coeliac disease
- Cow's milk intolerance

Giardia cysts may be detected in stool. An immunoassay is available to detect giardia antigen. More sensitive is the detection of trophozoites in duodenal aspirates or biopsy. The serum folate is usually normal or raised in bacterial overgrowth, and the iron level is not usually low.

Case 10.6

1. a
2. a

Ventricular septal rupture occurs most commonly after anterior MI. There is a bimodal incidence, with peaks on day one and days three to five. Cardiac output is commonly measured by thermodilution, with saline injected through the proximal port and the temperature measured at the distal end of the catheter. It thus measures right ventricular output. This is high on account of the ruptured septum. Immediate surgery is recommended after echocardiographic confirmation of the diagnosis, whatever the clinical status of the patient, as ruptures may suddenly increase in size. IABP, afterload reduction, diuretics and inotropes may temporize. Peripheral vasoconstriction with noradrenaline is likely to worsen the intracardiac shunt. (IABPs worsen aortic regurgitation due to increased diastolic pressure.)

Case 10.7

1. d
2. a

Bilateral livedo reticularis is shown. Livedo reticularis results from any disorder impeding drainage of superficial venules into the dermis. Embolism from endocarditis could cause this, but one would expect signs in the upper limbs. She has also had negative blood cultures. Cholesterol emboli result in small-vessel disease. This usually occurs in patients with atherosclerosis following arterial catheterization, but it may occur spontaneously or with warfarin. The kidneys and lower extremities are often affected selectively, but emboli may reach any abdominal organ, spinal cord, brain or retina, depending on the site of disrupted atheroma. Renal failure and a transient eosinophilia or eosinophiluria is common. Cholesterol emboli are often misdiagnosed but should be considered in the differential of a vasculitic illness, particularly in the elderly. The definitive diagnostic procedure is a renal biopsy, which shows needle-shaped clefts left by the cholesterol crystals that have dissolved during the specimen preparation. Treatment is supportive. Microscopic polyangiitis is a multisystem vasculitis that is usually ANCA-positive (70–80%). Eosinophilia is seen more commonly in Churg–Strauss syndrome, but this is less likely in the absence of lung pathology or asthma. The average eosinophilia in Churg–Strauss syndrome is $8 \times 10^9/l$, with most being greater than $1.5 \times 10^9/l$. A smaller eosinophilia may also be seen in classic PAN. Cryoglobulinaemia is an important differential, but in this classical scenario the marks go to cholesterol emboli.

Case 10.8

1. b
2. b

In subacute polymyositis, constitutional disturbance, muscle pain and tenderness are often absent, the clinical picture resembling a dystrophy. Occasionally, symptoms begin in one limb before becoming generalized. Neck muscles are often involved. Weakness may spread to involve respiratory muscles, resulting in ventilatory failure, and pharyngeal muscles, resulting in aspiration. Some patients exhibit Raynaud's phenomenon, joint pains or scleroderma-like skin plaques. Positive Jo-1 antibodies are a marker for the development of an associated alveolitis. Pulmonary hypertension occurs with scleroderma but not with myositis. The association between polymyositis and malignancy is weaker than that seen with dermatomyositis. PMR causes pain and stiffness predominant over weakness. There are no specific features to suggest a myositis secondary to any other connective tissue diseases. CK is a very useful marker for muscle disease but may be raised with muscular dystrophies and myopathies as well as with myositis.

Other forms of myositis (most are associated with pain) include:

*   Viruses (e.g. Coxsackie B, Bornholm disease)
*   Trichinosis
*   Parasitic and fungal infections (e.g. toxoplasmosis, cysticercosis)
*   Eosinophilic myositis (treat with steroids)
*   Granulomatous myositis (localized or part of generalized sarcoidosis)
*   Localized nodular myositis (painful muscle swellings)
*   Inclusion body myositis (older males, proximal and distal muscles, steroid-resistant)

Case 10.9

1. c
2. a

AION may be non-arteritic or arteritic in origin. The former is associated with hypertension and diabetes and often affects branch vessels, resulting in altitudinal defects. The latter may present suddenly without any preceding symptoms of giant cell arteritis. It usually affects the central vessels, wiping out vision completely. The diagnosis must be established urgently to try to save the fellow eye. ESR and/or CRP are usually, but not always, raised. Papilloedema is usually bilateral, and visual acuity is little affected. Papillitis (optic neuritis) does cause a loss of acuity but the disc is not pale acutely, although atrophy may follow. The field defect is a central scotoma. Pain is usual and is worse on eye movement.

Case 10.10

1. c

Laparotomy is necessary if decompressive sigmoidoscopy fails. Another 'obstruction' to remember is the distal intestinal obstruction syndrome (meconium ileus equivalent) in adult cystic fibrosis. Presentation is often with a palpable mass and dilated loops of small bowel on X-ray. Treatment is with intravenous fluids, high-dose pancreatic enzyme supplements, H_2 blockers and acetylcysteine. Also remember intestinal pseudo-obstruction with oesophageal reflux and steatorrhoea in systemic sclerosis.

Exam 11

Case 11.1

1. d, e

Images of a left apical lung tumour and digital clubbing are shown here. The scintigram description and clubbing are typical of HPOA, which occurs in 1–10% of patients with lung cancer and has a particular association with adenocarcinoma. Radiographically, it is classically seen as candle-wax thickening of the periosteum. Squamous cell carcinomas may release PTHrP, but pseudoclubbing and osteitis fibrosa cystica are generally seen only in very long-standing primary hyperparathyroidism. Small-cell carcinomas are associated with ADH or ACTH production, and also are the most common tumour type associated with sensory neuropathy (detected with neurophysiology in up to 50% of patients). A low rheumatoid titre is common in a 70-year-old. It would be much higher in somebody with nodules. Rheumatoid nodules do, however, pose a common diagnostic problem. Cavitation may lead to haemoptysis and concern about malignancy. Percutaneous needle aspiration is generally unrewarding and therefore open lung biopsy is necessary if tissue diagnosis is needed to exclude malignancy.

Case 11.2

2. f, h

Gitelman's syndrome is now thought to be one of the commonest causes of hypokalaemia in young patients taking no medication, with prevalence estimates of 20 per million from population studies. It is caused by mutations in the thiazide-sensitive Na/K transporter, such that the clinical syndrome resembles that of ingestion of thiazide diuretics, with hypomagnesaemia and hypocalciuria in addition to hypokalaemia. It manifests in reduced quality of life due to a range of subtle symptoms, including muscle stiffness and cramps, nocturia, fatigue and salt craving. Without molecular genetic testing, it is a diagnosis of exclusion, depending particularly on exclusion of abuse of laxatives or thiazide diuretics. The analogous Bartter's syndrome is caused by mutations of the Na/K/Cl loop-diuretic-sensitive channel, is not associated with hypocalciuria, and is generally apparent at a younger age due to failure to thrive and polyuria.

Hypokalaemic periodic paralysis is caused by calcium channel mutations. It is characterized by episodic paralysis starting before age 25 years, with hypokalaemia provoked after exercise or large meals. Prophylactic treatment is with potassium salts and acetazolamide.

The active principle of liquorice is glycyrrhizic acid, which inhibits 11-β-hydroxysteroid dehydrogenase and renders mineralocorticoid receptors susceptible to activation by cortisol, giving a hyperaldosteronism-like picture.

Case 11.3

1. b
2. b

Most patients' platelets have the A1 antigen. Those lacking it can develop anti-A1 antibodies from fetomaternal blood transfer or previous transfusion. The patient's own platelets, for unknown reasons, seem to be destroyed as well. Treatment is with A1-negative platelet transfusion, intravenous Ig or plasmapheresis.

Case 11.4

1. a
2. a, f

This man has likely nephrotic syndrome with anasarca and raised lipids. He may have had recurrent urinary tract infections, but chronic pyelonephritis does not cause the nephrotic syndrome per se. The JVP is not raised in uncomplicated nephrotic syndrome and therefore here suggests an additional pathology. Indeed, he has signs of predominantly right-sided restrictive heart failure. Moreover, he has easy bruising and macroglossia. This is all most consistent with AL amyloidosis (the most common systemic amyloidosis, with predilection for heart, kidneys, tongue and skin). Chronic pressure sores and pyelonephritis may result in systemic AA amyloidosis, but this does not produce macroglossia and affects the heart very rarely.

The ECG may show characteristic low voltages, conduction delay and pseudoinfarction pattern, while echocardiography would most likely reveal diastolic dysfunction with reversed E : A ratio and sparkling granular echotexture of the myocardium. Biopsy of multiple tissues (gingival, rectum, subcutaneous fat, heart, kidney) in conjunction with Congo red/polarized microscopy may make the diagnosis, but the rectum is used most commonly. Coagulopathy due to hepatic involvement makes care essential. A monoclonal Ig should be sought with electrophoresis of concentrated urine.

Case 11.5

1. c
2. c
3. a, d, e, f

She has a subacute cerebellar syndrome. CT scans are particularly inferior to MRI scans at picking up posterior fossa lesions, but one would expect to see any tumour with this degree of clinical severity. Her CT scan is normal (12, inter-hemispheric fissure; 13, lateral ventricles; 14, third ventricle; 15, sylvian fissure; 16, pineal gland; 17, quadrigeminal cistern; 18, vermis of cerebellum). She has no other features to suggest hypothyroidism, although this is a possibility. There is nothing to suggest that she has developed a nutritional deficiency or Wernicke's encephalopathy. Pure alcoholic cerebellar degeneration is primarily truncal. Anti-Yo and -Hu antibodies are paraneoplastic markers. Anti-Yo antibodies are present in half of paraneoplastic cerebellar degenerations and are especially associated with ovarian and breast carcinomas. Anti-Hu antibodies are associated more with small-cell carcinomas. Many other anti-neuronal paraneoplastic antibodies have been described more recently.

Other miscellaneous features of hypothyroidism include:

- Depression, somnolence and psychosis
- Weakness and muscle cramps
- Entrapment neuropathy and polyneuropathy
- Deafness
- Hypovolaemia and diastolic hypertension

Case 11.6

1. d
2. b

This patient has a low albumin. Liver function is otherwise normal (the slightly raised ALP is growth-related) and there is no urinary loss. She therefore must have a protein-losing enteropathy. There are many causes for loss of plasma proteins, including:

- Mucosal pathology
- Malignancy
- Crohn's disease
- Multiple ulcers
- Coeliac disease
- Tropical sprue
- Whipple's disease
- Menetrier's disease

- Lymphatic abnormalities
- Constrictive pericarditis
- Parasitic infection
- Tuberculosis
- Primary lymphangiectasia

The protein loss, together with the lymphopoenia, low immunoglobulin levels, mild steatorrhoea and normal radiology, make primary lymphangiectasia the most likely diagnosis. Presentation may occur at any time. The lymphatic abnormality may be primary or secondary to venous hypertension (e.g. constrictive pericarditis) or conditions such as SLE. The defect may be generalized, with lymphoedema and chylous ascites also present. Dilated lacteals are seen on biopsy. The immunoglobulin deficiency does not seem to lead to an excess of infections. Radiolabelled albumin studies would confirm a protein-losing enteropathy but not the specific cause. Medium-chain triglycerides do not need to be absorbed via the lymphatic system and therefore are an important part of treatment. There is some anecdotal evidence that octreotide may have marked benefits through a reduction in protein loss.

Case 11.7

1. d
2. e

Regular cannon waves are shown in this stretch of JVP recording. Independent atrial activity results in intermittent atrial contraction against a closed atrioventricular valve. This may lead to the triggering of vasodepressor reflexes, venous regurgitation and left ventricular underfilling, and can be seen as cannon waves in the JVP. Complete heart block leads to irregular cannon waves, junctional rhythms to regular cannon waves. Apart from maintaining AV synchrony with dual chamber pacing, benefit may also accrue from incorporating hysteresis into a VVI system, i.e. the rate at which pacing is triggered is set 15–20 bpm below the paced rate, making the chance of coincident atrial and ventricular contraction less.

Case 11.8

1. b
2. d, e

The catheter data are consistent with an ASD, 90% of which are of ostium secundum type. Characteristically, this results in an RSR' pattern in V1 with right axis deviation (left axis for ostium primum). With significant shunts, clinical signs result from high flow through the right-sided chambers and valves, with wide fixed splitting of S2.

Pulmonary plethora and a large right atrium may be seen on CXR, and with time right-sided pressure will equalize with the left as Eisenmenger's syndrome develops. Paradoxical embolism after transient high right-sided pressures, as seen in venous thromboembolism, may lead to CVAs.

Beware of dual diagnoses, e.g. Lutembacher's syndrome, the co-incidence of ASD and mitral stenosis (congenital, acquired through rheumatic fever with pre-existing ASD, iatrogenic following trans-septal valvuloplasty).

Case 11.9

1. b
2. a

Pituitary apoplexy refers to acute infarction of the pituitary. This is commonly due to the presence of a large tumour, in this case also causing Cushing's syndrome. Such tumours often do not present until the apoplectic attack if they are non-secretory. Other predisposing causes include postpartum hypotension (Sheehan's syndrome), raised intracranial pressure and systemic anticoagulation. The infarction and subsequent oedema, particularly if haemorrhagic in nature, results in compression of neighbouring structures. Hence, retro-orbital pain and ophthalmoplegia may develop. If the carotid artery is compressed, hemisphere signs may result. Meningeal irritation and coma occur if the subarachnoid space is involved. Urgent neurosurgical decompression may be necessary. Treatment for hypopituitarism should be started immediately with glucocorticoid. In the absence of clues to the diagnosis of a prior pituitary tumour, an intracranial aneurysm should be considered.

Case 11.10

1. c
2. b
3. b

Calcium oxalate deposits in the kidneys, heart conducting system and brain. Glycolate causes the high anion gap acidosis. The urine may fluoresce with Wood's light. Ethylene glycol has a half-life of three hours. Treatment is aimed at slowing down its metabolism to the toxic breakdown products by competitive inhibition of the enzymes with ethanol. The toxins can be removed by dialysis. Rhabdomyolysis would not produce such a profound acidosis with this degree of renal failure, and the phosphate would be raised. Also, the urine dipstick detected no myoglobin. Correcting metabolic and electrolyte disturbance is important but is included in the ICU general supportive care and thus receives fewer marks. A related case history would be of an alcoholic presenting with decreased visual acuity and raised anion gap metabolic acidosis from methanol poisoning. Other features of ethylene glycol poisoning include:

- Haematemesis
- Papilloedema
- Myoclonic jerks
- Cranial nerve palsies
- Cardiac failure
- Loin pain

Exam 12

Case 12.1

1. c

Bronchorrhoea (copious sputum) is the classical symptom of alveolar cell carcinoma but occurs in less than 20% of cases. Up to 1 l/day may be produced and can lead to respiratory failure. It is related less clearly than other tumours to smoking. Its peripheral origin means that bronchoscopy is often normal. The CXR appearance may also mimic pulmonary oedema, haemorrhage or alveolar proteinosis.

Case 12.2

1. a
2. e

A patient from the Far East with cholangitis, especially a chef, must be suspected of harbouring liver flukes. *Clonorchis sinensis* is the commonest in that part of the world, being acquired from poorly cooked fish. Worms are up to 2 cm long and can live in small to medium-sized bile ducts for up to 25 years. Other complications include cholelithiasis, pancreatitis and cholangiocarcinoma. Ova in the faeces are used for diagnosis. Treatment is with praziquantel.

Other conditions associated with acute cholangitis include:

*   Primary and secondary sclerosing cholangitis (rarely)
*   Caroli's disease (congenital intrahepatic biliary dilation)
*   Biliary enteric fistulae
*   Common bile duct stones
*   Benign strictures

Note that malignant strictures usually produce complete obstruction and hence the bile remains sterile.

Note: *Acanthamoeba* cause keratitis in contact-lens wearers, while *Paragonimus* species are lung-dwelling trematodes.

Case 12.3

1. f
2. d

Bone pain in anyone of African ancestry raises the possibility of sickle cell crisis. However, the patient is too old to be a homozygous new presentation and heterozygotes run into problems only with severe hypoxia, e.g. anaesthesia and very high altitude (although renal papillary necrosis due to high intramedullary osmolalities may occur). The low MCH and raised red cell count suggest thalassaemia trait. Therefore, the most likely diagnosis is sickle beta-thalassaemia leading to bilateral avascular necrosis of the femoral heads. Mediterranean sickle beta^0-thalassaemia often behaves like sickle cell anaemia, whereas African sickle beta$^+$-thalassaemia patients have a mild anaemia with occasional (or no) sickling episodes (0 refers to an absence of and + to a reduced production of the globin chain). Haemoglobin SC disease is another haemoglobinopathy; it may present in adult life, often with haematuria, aseptic necrosis, thrombosis and retinal vascular occlusion. Haemoglobin CC disease leads to anaemia with a characteristic blood film. Note that haemoglobin C beta^0-thalassaemia patients have a mild anaemia with splenomegaly, while the haemoglobin E thalassaemia seen in South-East Asia/India behaves like homozygous beta^0-thalassaemia. Sickle cell trait generally features 60% haemoglobin A and 40% haemoglobin S, although additional thalassaemia trait reverses this.

Note: remember *Salmonella* osteomyelitis in sickle cell anaemia and *Yersinia* infection in patients on desferrioxamine.

Case 12.4

1. e
2. a, h

TTP (aka Moschkowitz disease) classically presents as acute and fluctuating neurology in a young female associated with fever and renal impairment. Thrombocytopenia and microangiopathic haemolytic anaemia (MAHA) are seen on investigation. Unlike the situation seen in DIC, the PT and APTT are normal or prolonged only slightly. TTP may be inherited or acquired and in both cases is believed to be due to loss of von Willebrand factor-cleaving protease activity (either through loss of expression or blocking antibodies). A chronic, relapsing form is recognized. Septicaemic states with purpura would be expected to cause DIC together with hypotension rather than hypertension. If she had been pregnant, the HELLP (hypertension, elevated liver enzymes and low platelets) syndrome would have been a possible diagnosis.

Associations of HUS/TTP include:

- Pregnancy or postpartum state
- *Escherchia coli* O157/H7 or *Shigella* infection

- HIV
- Drugs (e.g. ticlopidine, clopidogrel, OCP, cyclosporin, mitomycin)
- Accelerated hypertension
- Tumours
- SLE

Case 12.5

1. a, e
2. a, h

A prolonged APTT could be due to an inhibitor (e.g. anticardiolipin antibody) or a factor deficiency (factors XII, XI, IX and VIII, prekallikrein and high-molecular-weight kininogen). Factor XII deficiency or lupus anticoagulant *in vivo* may be associated with thrombosis but not with bleeding. Factor XI deficiency is an incompletely penetrant autosomal recessive disorder that presents with relatively minor bleeding problems after surgery or trauma. It is associated with Noonan's syndrome. Prekallikrein and high-molecular-weight kininogen deficiency cause in vitro abnormalities of clotting tests but no in vivo bleeding problems. This leaves factor VIII and IX deficiencies. These are X-linked disorders with a spontaneous mutation rate of 30%. Haemophilia may occur in females in the following circumstances: if there is preferential inactivation of paternally inherited X chromosomes, if a male haemophiliac marries a female carrier, with genetic mosaicism, and in Turner's syndrome. This patient is aged 16 years, short and still prepubertal, and therefore Turner's syndrome is the most likely diagnosis.

Dilute Russell's viper venom testing is used as an additional test for lupus anticoagulant.

Case 12.6

1. e
2. a

Pneumatosis cystoides intestinalis refers to the presence of gas filled pseudocysts in the bowel wall (submucosal or subserosal). They may cause colicky pain, diarrhoea, tenesmus, bleeding and obstruction. The appearance of blue sessile polyps with normal overlying mucosa and multiple, discrete gas pockets on plain films is very characteristic. Puncture of the endoscopic lesions leads to deflation. The condition is a sign rather than a disease in itself, and it can be associated with multiple conditions, including instrumentation, COAD, necrotizing enterocolitis, ischaemic colitis, systemic sclerosis, pyloric stenosis and immunosuppression. In this case, it is likely to be idiopathic in association with COAD. The characteristic presence of pneumoperitoneum without signs of peritoneal irritation is a clue that surgery is not immediately necessary and should prompt a careful evaluation. The best treatment is high-concentration oxygen (caution if COAD). Hyperbaric oxygen may be necessary in resistant cases. Antibiotics to decrease gas-forming organisms have also been used. In this case, a double-contrast barium enema is shown, revealing characteristic gas-filled bubbles in the bowel wall.

Case 12.7

1. b, c

A murmur in systole and diastole in combination with a collapsing pulse and raised JVP suggests run-off from the left side of the heart to the right. If the murmur is truly continuous, then the history and examination are very suggestive of a ruptured sinus of Valsalva aneurysm. This is either a congenital anomaly caused by failure of fusion of the media of the aorta and aortic valve annulus fibrosis or an acquired defect in infective endocarditis. The aneurysm may rupture into the RV, RA, LV or pericardium, causing acute chest pain and breathlessness. If it ruptures into the right side of the heart, then the RV does not dilate as the rupture is acute and the RV does not have time to adapt. In the scenario of a right-sided rupture, the diagnosis is suggested by a step up in saturation in the pulmonary artery (good data interpretation question) and is confirmed by an aortic root angiogram. In practice, disintegration of part of the aortic valve may lead to a loud systolic and diastolic murmur, which could be confused with a continuous murmur, although a further pointer away from it in this case is the absence of pulmonary oedema.

Case 12.8

1. e

Exposed to cattle in sub-Saharan Africa at close quarters, this man may well have been exposed to anthrax spores in sufficient numbers to cause inhalational anthrax. This is characterized by an incubation period of around six days before non-specific symptoms appear, which could be consistent with a viral URTI. After two to three days, a second phase of the illness develops, with stridor, diaphoresis, abrupt dyspnoea and cyanosis, leading swiftly to cardiovascular collapse and death a mean of three days after the start of symptoms. Radiography reveals a characteristic symmetrically enlarged mediastinum due to haemorrhagic lymphadenitis and mediastinitis, which may be seen early in the illness. Although spores are deposited in the parenchyma of the lung, pulmonary infiltrates are uncommon, although pleural effusions may be seen. Mortality is 80–100% despite treatment with intravenous ciprofloxacin and a second agent such as penicillin or doxycycline. In this case, the exposure made the diagnosis relatively easy in conjunction with the clinical course, but in the present era of bioterrorism a high index of suspicion needs to be maintained by physicians even without this.

Ninety-five per cent of anthrax is cutaneous (classically a large black eschar surrounded by intense, gelatinous oedema – do not debride in case of bacteraemia), but gastrointestinal (from contaminated meat – dysentery, acute abdomen with haemorrhagic mesenteric lymphadenitis and 50% mortality) and meningeal (in context of bacteraemia) disease may also occur.

Case 12.9

1. b
2. d

Kallman's syndrome results from abnormal migration of the GnRH-secreting neurons that originate in the nasal placode. The olfactory neurones often suffer the same fate, with consequent anosmia (up to 50% of cases). Other associated defects include cleft palate, colour-blindness, nerve deafness, mirror movements, exostoses and unilateral renal agenesis. It may be sporadic, X-linked dominant or autosomal dominant, or recessive with variable penetrance, and there is a strong male preponderance. The most common mutation is in the KAL gene on the X chromosome. Anorexia, malabsorption and excessive exercise may all cause low LH and FSH. Hypogonadotrophic hypogonadism is also associated with the Prader–Willi and Laurence–Moon–Biedl/Bardet–Biedl syndromes and familial cerebellar ataxia, among others.

Case 12.10

1. d
2. a

Retinitis pigmentosa usually develops in the Kearnes–Sayre syndrome. Other features that may be present include short stature, diabetes, hypoparathyroidism, proximal muscle weakness and deafness. Myasthenia gravis may cause a non-fatiguable ptosis but would not explain the heart block. Other diagnoses to be considered in cases of ophthalmoplegia include thyroid eye disease, congenital myopathy and oculopharyngeal dystrophy (autosomal dominant with dysphagia).

Other mitochondrial syndromes include MERRF (myoclonic epilepsy with ragged red fibres), presenting with myoclonus, epilepsy and ataxia, and MELAS (mitochondrial encephalopathy, lactic acidosis and stroke-like illness), often presenting with migrainous prodrome followed by a focal seizure and then a stroke. Ophthalmoplegia, short stature, deafness and peripheral neuropathy may provide the clue.

Exam 13

████████████

Case 13.1

1. b
2. b, d, e, f
3. b

CFA refers most specifically to a histological picture of heterogeneous fibrosis on a background of chronic inflammation (aka idiopathic pulmonary fibrosis or usual interstitial pneumonia). There is, however, a spectrum of idiopathic pneumonias with different degrees of alveolar injury, cellularity and fibrosis. These include desquamative interstitial pneumonia, cryptogenic organizing pneumonia (COP)/bronchiolitis obliterans with organizing pneumonia (BOOP), diffuse alveolar damage and non-specific interstitial pneumonia. Patients with desquamative histology have a more favourable response to treatment. Before CFA can be diagnosed, history and examination are paramount in excluding the secondary causes of this picture:

• Extrinsic allergic alveolitis (chronic stage)
• Asbestosis/silicosis
• Drug therapy, e.g. cytotoxics, amiodarone, gold, phenytoin
• Inhaled agents (e.g. mercury vapour)
• Paraquat poisoning
• Irradiation

Fifty per cent of patients with CFA are clubbed. Weakly positive rheumatoid factor, ANA and raised inflammatory markers are found in up to 30%, and in occasional cases the CXR is normal despite histological proof and consistent clinical picture. Trials of therapy have been clouded by inconsistent case mixes and terminology, but there is little evidence for the efficacy of steroids for this particular pathology. They should thus be used with careful attention to any positive response. The prognosis is very poor, but unilateral lung transplantation has been used with some success.

Case 13.2

1. e

Tonsillar diphtheria can look like any other form of tonsillitis, although the adherent grey-brown membrane is quite distinctive and may extend on to the palate beyond the tonsils and be associated with very marked oedema ('bull neck'). Upper respiratory obstruction is one of the early perils. Ten per cent develop myocarditis from the first week and paralyses from the third week (palatal, double vision and loss of accommodation, laryngeal and pharyngeal paralyses are commonest). Treatment is with urgent hyperimmune horse serum (beware acute hypersensitivity and later serum sickness), penicillin or erythromycin to eradicate organisms and ICU/CCU for appropriate monitoring. Temporary pacing may be required for severe conduction abnormalities. Although extremely rare in well-immunized Western populations, the disease is a threat wherever coverage is poor, as evidenced recently in a huge surge in cases in the countries of the former Soviet Union immediately after its collapse.

Case 13.3

1. a
2. g

Anaemia and abdominal pain: ?PNH. Presentation is with insidious fatigue from chronic low-grade haemolysis, sometimes punctuated by paroxysms of haemolysis with visible haemoglobinuria. Patients become iron deficient. Thrombosis in small abdominal veins causes attacks of abdominal pain, but it is thrombosis elsewhere that causes the morbidity. There is a strong association with marrow hypoplasia. Patients are mildly jaundiced, sometimes with slight hepatosplenomegaly. Intrahepatic venous thrombosis causes the Budd–Chiari syndrome, with rapid liver enlargement and ascites. Also, remember renal vein thrombosis. The length of the illness, haemolysis and low ESR make metastatic disease less likely. The serology and ESR effectively exclude SLE. The molecular pathology of PNH is interesting, consisting of somatic mutation in a clone of red cell progenitors in the PIG-A gene, which synthesizes the GPI anchor for various plasma-membrane proteins. As these include molecules such as decay-accelerating factor, which damps down the ever-present threat of complement attack, cells without GPI-linked proteins are very susceptible to lysis by complement under stressed conditions. A hypoplastic marrow environment seems necessary to allow the clone to expand. This is the basis of Ham's test, which assays red cell stability in acidified serum. More modern testing includes electrophoresis of cell-surface proteins to look for those attached by GPI anchors.

Case 13.4

1. c
2. d

This storage disease may be relapsing and remitting or steadily progressive. Symptoms may get dramatically worse on dieting. Treatment is plasmapheresis, cessation of dieting and a chlorophyll-free diet. Other features may include:

- Retinitis pigmentosa
- Cardiomyopathy
- Epiphyseal dysplasia, e.g. short metacarpals, pes cavus
- Anosmia

Case 13.5

1. b

The CT scan shows bronchiectasis. Note the widened bronchi with thickened walls. In ataxia telangiectasia, patients are progressively ataxic from an early age, with oculomotor apraxia and choreoathetosis developing later. Inheritance is autosomal recessive. The clinical hallmark is the multiple telangiectasiae, seen particularly in the conjunctivae. Alpha-fetoprotein levels may be raised. Defects in cell and humoral immunity, particularly with IgA and IgE deficiency and defective DNA repair, result in recurrent infection and tumour susceptibility. Death in teens or twenties from bronchiectasis is typical.

Case 13.6

1. f
2. e

Chronic constrictive pericarditis is well known to present to gastroenterologists occasionally as cirrhosis; thus, always beware the patient with chronic liver disease and distended neck veins. In this case, the clinical findings are characteristic and the constriction is most likely related to previous cardiac surgery. The most important cardiac differential is restrictive cardiomyopathy, militated against in this case by the clinical context and third heart sound. Differentiation requires functional assessment with four-chamber catheterization, and saline infusion if necessary, to demonstrate characteristic pressure traces and normalization of pressure in all chambers in diastole. Functional MRI is also useful where available. Merely demonstrating a thickened pericardium is not diagnostic. The JVP may rise on inspiration (Kussmaul's sign), and the x and y descents are prominent. Pulsus paradoxus is not seen in constrictive pericarditis. Definitive treatment is surgical.

Other causes of constrictive pericarditis include:

- Idiopathic
- TB (or histoplasmosis rarely)

- Connective tissue disorders
- Sequel to acute suppurative pericarditis
- Malignancy
- Trauma
- Uraemia
- Radiation

Case 13.7

1. b
2. b, d

Idiopathic hypercalciuria is a common cause of stones. It is believed to result from dysregulated vitamin D action on the gut, bones or kidney. The common variant is due to increased intestinal calcium absorption, with a compensatory increase in urine calcium excretion (via low PTH). In this case, decreased dietary calcium is appropriate (to RDA of 1–1.2 g). A less common variant is due to calcium leakage through the tubules, PTH and vitamin D acting to normalize the blood calcium via increased absorption. Treatment is to decrease the leak by decreasing dietary sodium and protein, plus the use of thiazide diuretics and amiloride. Triamterene should be avoided, since it may precipitate and produce stones. A raised fluid intake will help in all forms of nephrolithiasis (aim to produce 2 l/day of urine, usually with 2–3 l intake). Medullary sponge kidney would be detected radiologically.

Other causes of normocalcaemic hypercalciuria include:

- General renal tubular dysfunction, e.g. Wilson's disease
- Distal renal tubular acidosis
- Sarcoidosis

Case 13.8

1. d
2. c

Takayasu's disease is due to a panarteritis of the aorta, its branches and the pulmonary artery. It is much more common in women than in men, and it is underdiagnosed. Symptoms wax and wane during the illness and change in character. There tends to be an initial inflammatory phase, with malaise, fever, arthralgia, stiff neck and joints, and transient neurological deficits. Sixty per cent of patients do not recall an inflammatory stage but present with the later complications of vascular narrowing and hypertension. Typical symptoms include leg and arm claudication, recurrent syncope and exertional breathlessness. Pulmonary hypertension may develop. Plain films may show aortic calcification, aneurysm formation or vascular pattern irregularity. The definitive investigation is, however, an angiogram of the entire aorta. Treatment is with steroids during the inflammatory stage and reconstructive vascular surgery/angioplasty as necessary when the inflammation has subsided. Mortality has been reported up to 75%, although latterly down to around 10%. Giant cell arteritis may have an aortitic component with claudication, but the disorder is very rare under the age of 50 and is rare without signs of temporal arteritis.

Case 13.9

1. d
2. c

If this were psychogenic polydipsia, then the plasma osmolality would not be raised and the weight would not fall so dramatically during water deprivation. Moreover, while medullary washout may decrease renal concentrating ability in polydipsia, it would not occur to this extent. To distinguish between the two forms of diabetes insipidus, a vasopressin analogue is administered. In equivocal cases, hypertonic saline infusion with serial osmolalities, ADH determination and a thirst chart may give a definitive result, but ADH assays are not widely available. The Ellsworth–Howard test is used to diagnose pseudohypoparathyroidism (urine cAMP response to intravenous PTH).

Causes of cranial diabetes insipidus include:

- Idiopathic
- Familial: autosomal dominant or in DIDMOAD (diabetes insipidus, diabetes mellitus, optic atrophy and deafness) syndrome
- Trauma/surgery
- Granulomatous disease
- Malignant infiltration
- Post-encephalitis/meningitis
- Aneurysm
- Pregnancy
- Autoimmune
- Hypophysitis
- Tumours

Causes of nephrogenic diabetes insipidus include:

- Familial (X-linked recessive or autosomal recessive)
- Idiopathic
- Hypercalcaemia
- Hypokalaemia

- Vascular disease, e.g. sickle cell anaemia
- Chronic renal disease
- Amyloidosis
- Myelomatosis
- Lithium
- Demeclocycline
- Amphotericin
- Glibenclamide

Case 13.10

1. c

The ECG shows 2 : 1 AV block with right bundle branch block. The non-conducted P waves are visible within the upstroke of the T wave. This, together with the rheumatological and neurological deficits, points towards Lyme disease. Not all patients remember being bitten and not all develop a rash. The cardiac, neurological and joint sequelae may occur in any order. Neurological involvement may be highly varied, although lymphocytic meningoradiculitis (Bannwarth's syndrome) is the most common manifestation in Europe.

Exam 14

Case 14.1

1. d
2. b

Complete the white cell count differential to reveal the eosinophilia. In conjunction with the abnormal CXR (bilateral upper-zone shadowing), the differential becomes that of a pulmonary eosinophilia:

- Fungal hypersensitivity:
  - *Aspergillus fumigatus* (80% in UK)
  - *Candida albicans*
- Helminthic infections
- Drug hypersensitivity: nitrofurantoin, aspirin, penicillin, imipramine, sulphonamides, etc.
- Vasculitis:
  - Wegener's
  - Churg–Strauss syndrome
  - PAN
- Cryptogenic (or chronic eosinophilic pneumonia)
- Hypereosinophilic syndrome
- Associated with lymphoma or carcinoma

There are no features in the history to suggest drugs as a cause, nor are there any clear features of malignancy. There were no specific clues to suggest Churg–Strauss syndrome (atopy, extrathoracic involvement) or Wegener's granulomatosis (sinusitis, renal involvement). In contrast to fungal and parasitic hypersensitivity, CPE patients have a relatively normal total IgE level with a disproportionately marked hypereosinophilia. Many have systemic features (malaise, weight loss, fever, raised ESR). Fifty per cent have asthmatic features. Hepatosplenomegaly and skin necrosis may develop when the disease begins to resemble Wegener's. When the disease is self-limiting, lasting less than one month, it is arbitrarily called Löffler's syndrome. The classic CXR appearance has been described as the photographic negative of the bat's wing shadows of pulmonary oedema. There is a prompt response to systemic steroids, which may need to be continued for one year. His sexual preferences were irrelevant.

Case 14.2

1. a, A
2. c, F
3. e, D
4. e, D
5. f, E

The estimated stool osmolality of $(2 \times Na) + (2 \times K)$ equals that measured. This is therefore a secretory diarrhoea. The corrected calcium is also high (this would need confirmation after rehydration). The commonest cause of secretory diarrhoea is infection, but most infections are relatively short-lived. Here, the history is long. In the absence of immunosuppression (and cryptosporidiosis), the most likely chronic infection would be giardiasis, although the diarrhoea is generally foul-smelling and associated with sulphurous eructation. Diagnosis is reached by microscopy of duodenal aspirate and biopsy and stool microscopy. Stool giardia immunoassay has a higher sensitivity than microscopy. Serum antibody estimation is less useful.

Next, one must consider laxative abuse. Psychological probing, urine screening and a locker search might therefore be appropriate. No marks are awarded for stool laxative testing, since this detects osmotic laxatives (e.g. Mg) and the diarrhoea is not osmotic. The appearance described in question 1 is that of melanosis coli, a common result of anthraquinone-containing laxative abuse.

A variety of endocrine causes should also be considered: VIPoma, carcinoid tumour, Zollinger–Ellison syndrome, medullary carcinoma of the thyroid and glucagonomas may all cause diarrhoea. All may be associated with raised calcium. In gastrinomas, the acid inactivates small-bowel enzymes, hence diarrhoea and steatorrhoea ensue, and may predate ulceration by many months. They are the commonest islet cell tumours in MEN1 after the age of 40 years (before this, insulinomas are more common). VIPomas cause large-volume diarrhoea without steatorrhoea. A marked acidosis may develop (this will partially mask the potassium deficiency). Patients presenting with circulatory shock should therefore have appropriate fluid resuscitation. Most gastrinomas and VIPomas have metastasized by the time of presentation and will be detected by ultrasound, CT, MRI or angiography. Most patients with medullary thyroid carcinoma (the *sine qua non* of MEN2, due to *ret* mutation) have a palpable neck mass. Severe diarrhoea may occur, and, if ACTH is secreted, Cushing's syndrome may also result. There is also a well-recognized association in MEN2A with lichen amyloidosis, appearing as pruritic plaques on the upper trunk and confirmed histologically.

For the record, somatostatinomas present with the triad of cholelithiasis, diabetes and steatorrhoea. Fifty per cent are associated with neurofibromatosis type 1. Glucagonomas present with a necrolytic migratory erythema, characteristically starting in the groin and sometimes involving mucous membranes (e.g. glossitis). Associated features include venous thrombosis, nail dystrophy, impaired glucose tolerance, bowel disturbance and neurological paraneoplastic syndromes. Pancreatic polypeptide is raised non-specifically with many gut hormone tumours.

Case 14.3

1. d

The preservation of the pupillary reflexes suggests the anatomical site of the pathology is beyond the midbrain, i.e. optic radiation or cortex. The macular sparing indicates that this is cortical. The acuteness of the onset suggests a vascular cause. The basilar artery gives rise to both posterior cerebral arteries, so thromboembolic basilar disease may lead to bilateral occipital infarcts. If the mesial temporal lobes are also involved, then memory disturbance will result (the confused, blind patient).

In hysteria, the area of field of vision usually remains the same when tested further away from the patient, defying light travelling in a straight line.

Case 14.4

1. d
2. e

Drug-induced lupus usually presents with fever, rash and serositis. Neurological and renal involvement is rare. The most predictable culprits are procainamide and hydralazine, with susceptibility determined in part by acetylation status of the patient. Thirty per cent of patients taking hydralazine become ANA-positive, of whom about 10% develop clinical features. Anti-histone antibodies are found in most patients, while anti-dsDNA antibodies are rare. On stopping the drug, symptoms settle spontaneously or with a short course of steroids over six months, although ANA positivity may persist for years.

Other drugs that may be implicated include:

- Phenytoin
- Procainamide
- Chlorpromazine
- Penicillin
- Tetracycline
- Griseofulvin
- Streptomycin
- Methyldopa

Case 14.5

1. a, b

This question is fair game for the adult MRCP section. The negative investigations exclude en masse most causes of seizures, including specific paediatric conditions.

Also, metabolic causes would not get better. This, together with basic pharmacology, leads you to the diagnosis. Heroin and methadone are the commonest drugs implicated, although most drugs of abuse can cause a similar picture. Benign familial convulsions is a rare autosomal dominant condition presenting with convulsions in the first three weeks of life and resolving spontaneously. (Pyridoxine dependency is an autosomal trait presenting with intractable seizures until large doses of pyridoxine are given, as was the case here.)

Case 14.6

1. d
2. b

This man has moderately severe leptospirosis, with characteristic conjunctival suffusion, severe muscle aches and frontal headache. Although typhoid, rickettsial disease, relapsing fevers and malaria enter the differential diagnosis, he has not left the UK. He is still in the septicaemic phase. These symptoms abate and immune symptoms develop, with the appearance of antibodies during the second week. Urine culture becomes positive in week two. Leptospires may, however, be seen in blood and CSF in week one. In practice, this organism is quite difficult to culture; most laboratories are unable to do this and so diagnosis relies on serology. The risk of Weil's disease is only around 10% in leptospirosis. Treatment is usually with a penicillin and/or macrolide, and Jarisch–Herxheimer reactions are rare (unlike relapsing fevers on treatment). Even in Weil's disease, liver failure is not common despite intense jaundice.

Case 14.7

1. a, e

The picture shows a large rheumatoid nodule. Possible causes of splenomegaly linked to rheumatoid arthritis are Felty's syndrome, AA amyloidosis, and cirrhosis with portal hypertension due to agents such as methotrexate. Felty's syndrome is a rare complication of long-standing rheumatoid arthritis. It is characterized by splenomegaly and leucopenia, and is often accompanied by lymphadenopathy, anaemia, thrombocytopenia, vasculitic ulcers and pigmentation.

Case 14.8

1. b, c
2. c

This lady gives a typical history for the relapsing and remitting form of MS. There is nothing in the history or examination to suggest a mimicking disease, such as sarcoidosis, Behçet's or Lyme disease, an AVM or a hereditary degenerative disorder. However, she has now developed lower motor neuron signs in the upper limbs. This is certainly completely consistent with MS, for if a demyelinating plaque lies adjacent to the dorsal root entry zone, then lower motor neuron signs will result. However, any neurological patient with long-standing spasticity or abnormal movements of the neck is also more prone to developing a cervical myelopathy. The resultant signs are often then dismissed as being due to the underlying disorder. Therefore, the important investigation is MRI of the cervical cord to exclude this.

Case 14.9

1. b

Pubic and axillary hair is diminished in hypopituitarism and hypogonadism but preserved in anorexia nervosa. Fine lanugo hair is characteristic of anorexia nervosa (shown here). Other clinical findings include low blood pressure and pulse, cool peripheries with dependent oedema, and fine, thin, dry skin. Complications include severe hypoglycaemia, which may go unnoticed on account of diminished sympathetic responses, and acute gastric dilation due to over-vigorous refeeding.

Endocrine features of anorexia nervosa include:

- Decreased conversion of T_4 to T_3 (some features of hypothyroidism may be present)
- Raised GH and cortisol levels, with loss of diurnal rhythm (stress/starvation response)
- Normal prolactin
- Electrolyte abnormalities (diuretic and laxative abuse)
- Raised cholesterol
- Raised beta-carotene
- Prepubertal LH and FSH, with low oestrogen and progesterone
- Impaired LH response to LH-releasing hormone

Case 14.10

1. c

He has an endophthalmitis and hypopyon. The cells and debris in the vitreous are obscuring direct ophthalmoscopy. In panophthalmitis, the sclera and cornea are inflamed. In endophthalmitis, the outer layers are affected only minimally. Causes are divided into suppurative and non-suppurative. Non-suppurative causes are many and include both primary ocular and systemic autoimmune disease, systemic infection with autoimmune ocular reaction (e.g. tuberculosis) and miscellaneous conditions such as sarcoidosis. However, infection is the diagnosis to exclude here, particularly with an obvious infective source, and therefore gains the marks. Fungi enter into the differential.

Exam 15

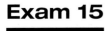

Case 15.1

1. a, d, e
2. d

Courvoisier's law states that jaundice in the presence of a palpable gallbladder is unlikely to be due to gallstones (rationalized by saying that gallstones result in either chronic inflammation or muscular hypertrophy, which makes the gallbladder less likely to dilate). The exception is concurrent obstruction by one stone in the common bile duct and another in the cystic duct. This picture may also be due, given appropriate exposure, to a liver fluke residing in the biliary tree (e.g. *Clonorchis sinensis*). In this case, the absence of abdominal pain and weight loss suggests that the pancreatic carcinoma is localized to the head of the pancreas. Pain, which is fairly common, suggests invasion retroperitoneally and of the splanchnic nerves. In 50% of cases the gallbladder is palpable (Courvoisier's sign). Ultrasound is the first-line investigation.

Other presentations of carcinoma of the pancreas include:

- Splenomegaly (portal vein compression)
- Polyarthritis
- Metastatic fat necrosis
- Upper gastrointestinal haemorrhage
- Migratory thrombophlebitis or thromboembolism
- Unexplained upper abdominal or back pain
- Acute pancreatitis in the older age group
- Sudden-onset diabetes when slim and with no family history
- Unexplained fever or weight loss

Case 15.2

1. a

Sorry: not all sewage workers have Weil's disease! Following a scratch, lick or cat bite, regional lymphadenitis develops, with microabscesses or granulomas on biopsy.

Most patients are only mildly unwell, but encephalitis, retinitis, hepatosplenomegaly and rashes may develop. When causing an eyelid or conjunctival granuloma in conjunction with preauricular lymphadenitis, it is termed Parinaud's oculoglandular syndrome. The bacterium is *Bartonella* (formerly *Rochalimaea*) *henselae*. Serological tests are available. Spontaneous resolution is the norm. The cat does not need to be killed, since they are infectious probably only for a short time.

Case 15.3

1. c
2. d

This patient has an eosinophilia. The picture is classic trichinosis. This is endemic throughout much of the pork-eating world but also in populations eating polar-bear meat. A mild gastroenteritis occurs as the larvae are liberated from their cysts by gastric juices. One week later muscles are invaded. Fever, myalgia and weakness of any muscles may be seen, but ocular, tongue, diaphragm, larynx and axial muscles are particularly affected. Eyelid and conjunctival oedema is common. The heart may be involved. Serology will not be positive until the larvae begin to encyst and calcify several weeks later. Note that given a case of unilateral proptosis in an otherwise well patient with no other signs, then the most likely diagnosis is euthyroid Grave's disease, demanding investigation with orbital CT and anti-thyroglobulin and microsomal antibodies. However, here Grave's disease would not explain the tongue weakness or eosinophilia and the onset would be slower.

Case 15.4

1. e, g

Diarrhoea persisting whilst nil by mouth suggests a secretory cause. The most likely cause is laxative abuse, but an endocrine tumour must be excluded. In fact, laxative abuse is thought to account for 4% of new out-patient gastroenterology referrals for evaluation of chronic diarrhoea and up to 20% in tertiary centres. There are five categories of patients with laxative-related factitious diarrhoea: (i) patients with eating disorders, including anorexia nervosa and bulimia; (ii) hysterical patients; (iii) patients driven by emotional problems; (iv) patients with Munchausen's syndrome; and (v) children who are abused by being given laxatives (the so-called Polle syndrome). Diagnostic testing is generally under-requested but should include urine alkalinization and thin-layer chromatography.

Features of laxative abuse include:

• Hypokalaemia
• Metabolic alkalosis

- Clubbing
- Diarrhoea whilst nil by mouth
- Loss of haustral pattern on barium enema but relatively normal macroscopic appearance
- Pigmentation of colonic mucosa (anthracenes, e.g. senna) and sometimes skin
- Pseudostrictures from spasm lasting hours
- Raised stool magnesium (osmotic laxatives)
- Uric acid kidney stones
- Osteomalacia
- Protein-losing enteropathy

Somatostatinomas are exceedingly rare, and are characterized by the triad of cholelithiasis, steatorrhoea and diabetes.

Case 15.5

1. d

There are three clues in the history: (i) salt wasting implies tubulointerstitial disease or chronic obstruction; (ii) intrinsic renal disease does not cause enough bleeding to cause a clot: what the patient thought was a clot could have been a stone or, more likely, a sloughed papilla; (iii) the history of headaches seals the link between points i and ii.

Note: If the history gives a late deterioration – ?transitional cell carcinoma of the renal pelvis. CT may be of help in detecting papillary calcification, which is one of the hallmarks of this condition.

Causes of salt-wasting nephritis include:

- Chronic pyelonephritis
- Myeloma
- Analgesic nephropathy
- Polycystic disease
- Heavy-metal poisoning
- Obstructive renal failure

Causes of papillary necrosis and shedding include:

- Diabetes mellitus
- Sickle cell disease
- Analgesic nephropathy
- Macroglobulinaemia
- Tuberculosis
- Acute pyelonephritis
- Profound hypotension

Case 15.6

1. d

Patients often present with band-like pain, which may radiate into the buttocks and thighs. Obstruction to the IVC or testicular vein may result in leg oedema or a hydrocoele. The classic description is of ureters pulled medially, but this may be a normal finding. CT may show a periaortic mass, but tissue should be obtained to exclude a lymphoma or carcinoma. The disease may be unilateral. In some cases, it is hypothesized to be due to an autoimmune reaction to material leaking from an atheromatous aorta. The idiopathic condition is associated with idiopathic mediastinal fibrosis, Riedel's thyroiditis, pseudotumour of the orbit and sclerosing cholangitis.

Causes of secondary retroperitoneal fibrosis include:

- Methysergide
- Ergot alkaloids
- Beta-blockers
- Bromocriptine
- Carcinoid tumours or carcinoma with desmoplastic reactions
- Radiation therapy
- Haemorrhage
- Infection (e.g. gonorrhoea)
- Sarcoidosis

Case 15.7

1. f

The first step is to localize the lesion anatomically. The flaccid quadriplegia could be due to an acute peripheral lesion (e.g. Guillain–Barré syndrome, porphyria, myasthenia gravis) or an acute central lesion. The evolution of upper motor neuron signs means that the lesion must be central. There are no signs of a lesion above the pons. The signs are symmetrical, with relative preservation of sensation and awareness, i.e. she is locked in. The lesion must be in the central pons. A vascular event would be likely to be asymmetrical and involve more lateral structures. MS demyelination may produce a locked-in state but rarely in the absence of previous history or other signs. The history of preceding severe dehydration with rapid resuscitation clinches the diagnosis. Any severe general medical condition followed by the development of quadriplegia and a pseudobulbar palsy should raise the possibility of central pontine myelinolysis. Severe hyponatraemia is often present. Very high serum osmolality is another implicated factor, e.g. in burns patients. Alcoholism is a common association.

Case 15.8

1. a, d
2. c, f

Causes of hyperphosphataemia include renal failure, rhabdomyolysis, hypoparathyroidism and pseudohypoparathyroidism. The latter is due to resistance of various end-organ tissues:

Type 1a patients have short stature, short metacarpals and other skeletal abnormalities, known as Albright's hereditary osteodystrophy, as well as calcium and phosphate abnormalities. There is often resistance to other hormones, such as TSH and gonadotrophins, and obesity.

Type 1b (as in this case) patients have only calcium and phosphate abnormalities, due to the same underlying mutation but inherited from their father, inducing tissue-specific gene-silencing. Bone is still susceptible to PTH activity and so ALP may be raised.

In both types 1a and 1b, neither urine cAMP nor urine phosphate rise following a PTH challenge.

Type 2 patients have only calcium and phosphate abnormalities, but only the urinary phosphorous excretion fails to respond to PTH.

Pseudopseudohypoparathyroidism refers to the skeletal abnormalities without calcium/phosphate derangement.

Note that a low serum magnesium will most commonly suppress PTH release and mimic hypoparathyroidism, but severe hypomagnesaemia may also result in PTH resistance and elevated PTH, with hypocalcaemia. Vitamin D deficiency classically produces both low calcium and low phosphate, but a normal circulating level of vitamin D should nonetheless be documented.

Treatment of pseudohypoparathyroidism is with activated vitamin D (calcitriol or 1-alpha-calcidol) to normalize calcium and PTH levels (the latter is important, as bone is not resistant to PTH in pseudohypoparathyroidism type 1b, putting the patient at risk of osteitis fibrosa cystica unless PTH is normalized).

Hypoparathyroidism may also form part of the DiGeorge syndrome (thymus aplasia results in predisposition to viral infection and autoimmune disease) or Gorlin's syndrome (palmar pits, bifid ribs, dental cysts, hypertelorism and basal cell carcinoma).

Case 15.9

1. b, d
2. c, i

Around 95% of hirsutism is caused by PCOS, which is most commonly gradually progressive and exacerbated by weight gain. The key features that aid triage of newly presenting patients with hirsutism are signs and symptoms of virilization, late onset and a short history, signs of Cushing's syndrome, and a testosterone level greater than 5 nM. However, the clinical suspicion is of paramount importance, as the testosterone cut-off is neither fully sensitive nor specific. These features should lead to a rapid work-up for possible virilizing tumours, which, although rare, carry a poor prognosis. Dehydroepiandrosterone sulphate (DHEAS), derived almost solely adrenally, may provide a clue of adrenal origin if grossly elevated, as may elevated urinary free cortisol.

Non-classical CAH may be picked up late but results most commonly in premature pubarche or a peripubertal onset of symptoms. There is no salt wasting. There will be a disproportionate rise in 17-hydroxyprogesterone with synacthen. All the steroid levels will be suppressed with dexamethasone (N.B. androgens and cortisol are measured). If they do not, then a tumour should be suspected and imaging of the ovaries and adrenals undertaken.

The figure below shows the mechanism of CAH:

Progesterone → *17OH* → 17-*OH* progesterone → Androgens

↓   ↓

↓ *21OH*   ↓ *21OH*

↓   ↓

11-Deoxycorticosterone   ↓

↓   ↓

↓ *11OH*   ↓ *11OH*

↓   ↓

Aldosterone   Cortisol

The keys to understanding the congenital adrenal hyperplasias are:

- Any blockage will cause synthesis to be increased in the other pathways
- 11-Deoxycorticosterone behaves like aldosterone; therefore:
  - 11-OH deficiency causes a build-up of 11-deoxycorticosterone, which causes hypertension and hypokalaemia with low renin levels. The increased androgen causes virilization
  - 17-OH deficiency prevents androgen formation and thus males are feminized. Females will be hypogonadal. The low cortisol may cause hypoglycaemia and the raised aldosterone hypertension and hypokalaemia with low renin levels
  - Total 21-OH deficiency blocks both aldosterone and 11-deoxycorticosterone production, with consequent salt wasting at birth. Females are virilized

Partial 21-OH deficiency causes increased synthesis through all pathways. Enough aldosterone is therefore produced to prevent salt wasting, but as a consequence excess androgens are produced.

Case 15.10

1. d

The normal plasma osmolality suggests that the low measured sodium is due to pseudohyponatraemia because of excess lipid or protein. Calculated osmolality is approximately 2[Na] + [urea] + [glucose]. Gaps greater than 10 mosmol/l suggest the presence of an excess of an osmotically active substance. In this case, a paraprotein is likely (not detected by urine dipstick). If paraprotein production were complicated by AL amyloidosis, then heavy proteinuria may result, which would be detected by conventional urinalysis. Note that in pseudohyponatraemia due to hyperglycaemia, in which water is drawn osmotically out of cells, the plasma osmolality will be raised.

Exam 16

Case 16.1

1. c
2. c

There are two diagnostic handles here: the effusion and the upper-zone shadowing. Rheumatoid effusions are unusual in the young and are typically small and asymptomatic. Systemic symptoms thus suggest secondary infection. This lady may well have rheumatoid disease, but this can only be ascribed as the cause of the effusion by exclusion. Although not diagnostic, there are characteristic features of the effusion. Lymphocyte predominance suggests TB, lymphoma or carcinoma, whereas neutrophil predominance is typical of rheumatoid. Low glucose content suggests rheumatoid, infection or malignancy. (Note, for reference, that eosinophils in pleural fluid are usually benign and non-diagnostic.)

The fibrotic upper-zone changes are typical of post-primary TB. This is a serious disease that should not be missed and hence gets the marks. Sarcoidosis, extrinsic allergic alveolitis and pneumoconiosis could mimic the fibrotic changes, but only sarcoidosis may cause a pleural effusion, although these are exceptionally rare, small and lymphocyte predominant. Upper-zone fibrosis in sarcoidosis is an end-stage occurrence.

Pleural biopsy will detect tuberculous granulomata in 80% of cases. Bronchoscopy would be reasonable here as the patient is sputum-negative. Tuberculin testing is highly suggestive but not diagnostic. A therapeutic trial of anti-tuberculous chemotherapy is sometimes necessary if no bacilli are seen or grown. Corticosteroids are often administered to reduce the size of the effusion and limit future scarring. A positive rheumatoid factor would not alter management.

Culture of pleural aspirate for mycobacteria would be an important further step, while thoracoscopic biopsy offers an alternative approach to an early tissue diagnosis.

Case 16.2

1. f

Vibrio vulnificus is a remarkably invasive organism that invades the intestinal lymphatics to cause septicaemia. It is usually contracted from contaminated seafood and is the commonest cause of severe *Vibrio* infections in the USA. Patients with liver disease are particularly predisposed to septicaemia, and in such patients the mortality is around 50%. Presentation is after 16 hours, with rapidly evolving septic shock. The lower extremity bullous rash after 36 hours is highly suggestive of the diagnosis. Patients with liver disease should thus be warned of the potential dangers of raw seafood. Healthy people with no underlying disease may develop otitis externa or wound infections from the same organism after swimming in the warm salt water of the American Gulf. Tetracycline, sometimes with gentamicin, is the treatment of choice. Despite the apparent obscurity of the question, much can be deduced from common sense and less abstruse knowledge: *V. cholerae* is the classical motile, curved, Gram-negative bacillus. However, shock in cholera is due to hypovolaemia rather than sepsis (as indicated by invasive monitoring here). However, this syndrome might be due to a related bacteria. *V. parahaemolyticus* is an important cause of gastroenteritis worldwide, particularly in Japan and the eastern USA. It is acquired from seafood; it most commonly produces a self-limiting watery diarrhoea after four hours to four days and lasts for three days.

Case 16.3

1. f
2. a

The Pagetic appearance of this woman's skull, characteristic distal femoral location of the swelling and pain, and the high ALP all suggest that she has long-standing Paget's disease complicated by osteosarcoma (osteolytic in this context on plain radiograph). This feared complication occurs in around 1% of those with Paget's disease (probably higher in polyostotic disease) and carries a poor prognosis (much worse than childhood osteosarcoma). Bone biopsy, MRI and/or CT are key investigations. Although ALP may rise explosively on malignant transformation, it may be elevated only mildly.

Other features/complications of Paget's disease include:

- Angioid streaks
- Hearing loss (otosclerosis and/or compression of VIII)
- Platybasia with brainstem compression
- Spinal cord compression
- Pathological fractures
- High-output heart failure
- Urolithiasis

Case 16.4

1. d

This is an example of Plummer–Vinson syndrome/Patterson–Brown–Kelly syndrome. The Crohn's disease has not been active enough to result in an associated malignancy or stricture. The clinical picture is of iron deficiency. It is a long history and she is quite well for a patient with a neoplasm. Therefore, a hypopharyngeal web is the most likely unifying diagnosis. A malignancy would need excluding and an underlying cause for the anaemia investigating. It is doubtful how significant this syndrome is as an entity in itself. The appearance on barium swallow of a post-cricoid web is shown below:

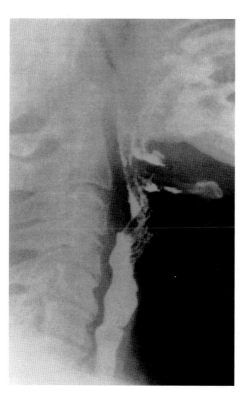

Case 16.5

1. c
2. g

The radiograph is normal. This patient has the nephrotic syndrome. In itself, this may cause abdominal pain through bowel-wall oedema. However, the localization of the pain means that renal-vein thrombosis due to this pro-thrombotic state must be considered. Also, remember that the associated hyperlipidaemia may cause acute pancreatitis. In adults idiopathic nephrotic syndrome is caused most commonly by membranous glomerulonephritis (30–40%), while in childhood the commonest cause is minimal-change nephropathy. As many as 50% of cases of nephrotic syndrome due to membranous glomerulonephritis are complicated by renal-vein thrombosis, which presents acutely as abdominal/flank pain, haematuria, left-sided varicocoele (remember the drainage of the left testicular vein to the left renal vein) and sudden fall in GFR. The chronic form may be asymptomatic. Most membranous glomerulonephritis is idiopathic, but also remember the well-established causes (grouped broadly as infections, systemic autoimmune disease, neoplasia, drugs and miscellaneous).

Case 16.6

1. c

post

Oxytocin is synthesized in the anterior pituitary with ADH, to which it has a similar structure. It may cause an ADH-like syndrome. Patients should not therefore receive large infusion volumes, in particular of dextrose, and they may need to be fluid-restricted. Oxytocin may also cause hypertension, subarachnoid haemorrhage and arrhythmias.

Case 16.7

1. c
2. d

The first step, as ever, is to localize the anatomy. This is upper motor neuron. The flaccidity reflects the acuteness of the illness. Bilateral foot weakness with up-going plantars may be due to a parasagittal lesion on account of the motor cortex representing the foot lying medially. However, here the extent of the weakness and clear sensory level locates the lesion to the spinal cord. The cause of the lesion may be extramedullary or intramedullary. Note that sacral fibres run on the outside of the cord, so sacral sparing often suggests an intramedullary lesion. Urgent imaging is always required to exclude extramedullary compressive lesions, here in particular an expanding haematoma.

Possible intramedullary causes, which would enter the differential, include tumour, vascular malformations and myelitis. Fifty per cent of cases of myelitis are related to infection, particularly viral (e.g. EBV, HIV). Other associations include sarcoidosis, paraneoplastic, autoimmune disorders, vaccination and surgery. Evolution is typically over days but may be over minutes or weeks. It is rarely the presenting feature of MS. CSF may be normal or have a raised protein or white cell count. Infectious causes include Lyme disease, syphilis and HIV. An anterior spinal artery thrombosis would be of more sudden onset and spare the posterior third of the cord, i.e. vibration and proprioception function.

Case 16.8

1. d
2. b
3. c, d, h

The CT is normal (12, inter-hemispheric fissure; 13, lateral ventricles; 16, pineal; 19, thalamus; 20, pathway of pyramidal tract; 21, caudate; 22, occipital horn of lateral ventricle).

A lymphocyte predominance is a feature of *Listeria*, although it may also occur in early bacterial infection and TB meningitis. *Listeria* usually causes a meningitis or brainstem meningoencephalitis, but it may cause a focal encephalitis with a normal CSF or multiple brain abscesses. Acute brainstem signs plus fever – ?*Listeria*. It is common in immunosuppressed and debilitated patients. Indeed, it is the commonest form of meningitis in transplant patients. Its importance lies in its resistance to cephalosporins. Ampicillin with or without gentamicin (not gentamicin in pregnancy) is usually used. Co-trimoxazole and chloramphenicol are alternatives.

CSF glucose is normally around half the value of the blood glucose. It is not corrected for cell count. It is the CSF protein level that is corrected against the CSF red cell count (1000 red cells = 0.1 g/dl protein).

Low CSF glucose + lymphocytes – think TB meningitis or *Listeria*.

Case 16.9

1. a, c, f
2. a, d, g

During transient global amnesia, the patient is able to perform complicated tasks but displays anterograde and, to a lesser extent, retrograde amnesia. An attack usually lasts hours, after which there is a complete recovery. It is idiopathic and has a good prognosis. Most patients have only one attack. The alertness and capability of performing complex tasks, e.g. shopping and driving, makes complex partial epilepsy less likely, but it still needs to be considered. Hypoglycaemic attacks, e.g. due to an insulinoma, are usually shorter-lasting and associated with adrenergic features. Psychogenic amnesia enters the differential but would be very unlikely to present so late in life. A conventional TIA would be unlikely to cause such long-lasting amnesia in isolation.

Causes of sudden-onset amnesia (with no, gradual or incomplete recovery) include:

* Bilateral hippocampal infarction
* Basal forebrain infarction

- Subarachnoid haemorrhage
- Carbon monoxide poisoning
- Trauma

Causes of subacute amnesia include:

- Wernicke–Korsakoff syndrome
- Herpes simplex encephalitis
- Granulomatous meningitides

Causes of slow-onset amnesia include:

- Limbic/third-ventricle tumours
- Degenerative disease, e.g. Alzheimer's

Case 16.10

1. c

This is a rare ectodermal syndrome worth including for its distinctive features. An enteropathy such as coeliac disease with severe vitamin deficiency is possible, but none of the common oral features of vitamin deficiency are present. Remember, also, that the spectrum of familial adenomatous polyposis includes Gardener's syndrome, with mesodermal tumours such as osteomas and sebaceous cysts. Screening for Gardener's syndrome may be with either gene probes or slit-lamp examination to look for pigmented retinal patches (congenital hypertrophy of the retinal pigment epithelium, CHRPE). Turcot's syndrome is the association of familial adenomatous polyposis with brain tumours. Peutz–Jeghers syndrome is spotty periorbital and sometimes digital pigmentation with small-bowel hamartomata. The main features of abetalipoproteinaemia (Bassen–Kornzweig disease) are steatorrhoea, ataxia, neuropathy, retinitis pigmentosa and acanthocytosis. Polyglandular autoimmune syndrome type 1 is characterized by mucocutaneous candidiasis, ectodermal dysplasia, hypoparathyroidism and adrenal insufficiency.

Exam 17

▬▬▬▬▬

Case 17.1

1. c
2. a

Diabetes is the commonest cause of Charcot neuroarthropathy, which often is triggered by trauma. It is not always painless, and it occurs particularly in feet with preserved blood flow but sensorimotor neuropathy and sympathetic denervation. It has several similarities to reflex sympathetic dystrophy. The first phase is an active process characterized by hyperaemia and increased bone resorption. This leads later to microfractures and ultimately foot deformity, which predisposes to further damage by introducing pressure points. There is some evidence that bisphosphonate infusions in the active stage of Charcot's neuroarthropathy may reduce bone remodelling, but the central plank of management is complete offloading of the foot, ideally with a total contact cast, until the hyperaemia has settled. Osteomyelitis underlying diabetic foot ulcers may be devoid of systemic signs or inflammatory response, and distinguishing it from a Charcot foot in that setting can be demanding, often requiring MRI or a combination of white cell and bone scintigraphy.

Case 17.2

1. e
2. a

The (limited) histological description is of a chronic active hepatitis. Most causes appear to have been excluded. However, a confounding factor is the transplant-related immunosuppression, which may prevent a detectable antibody response to HCV; hence, an antigen test is needed. Hepatitis C is an RNA virus, but detection is possible with the use of a reverse transcriptase and PCR. The raised MCV could simply reflect azathioprine use rather than alcohol abuse. An alternative diagnosis based on the clinical scenario if this patient were taking azathioprine would be aza-thioprine-induced hepatic veno-occlusive disease, which should be detected early and the azathioprine substituted by, for example mycophenolate mofetil, as it may otherwise be fatal. Histopathological features in this case are of sinusoidal congestion and centrilobular hepatocellular degeneration. (N.B. HBV is a DNA virus!)

Case 17.3

1. d, i
2. e

Melaena suggests haemorrhage proximal to the right side of the colon. Small-bowel follow-through may miss small structural lesions and vascular malformations. Angiodysplasia is associated with Turner's syndrome and aortic stenosis. (Angiodysplasia plus aortic stenosis is called Heyde's syndrome.) Up to 15% of patients with Turner's syndrome have bicuspid aortic valves, while up to 33% have renal abnormalities. Multiple pigmented naevi are a common cosmetic feature of the syndrome. Note that angiography cannot be carried out after barium studies. Around 30–50% of all patients with Turner's syndrome have a mosaic chromosomal complement (e.g. 45, X/46, XX). Meckel's diverticula can bleed due to ulceration in heterotopic gastric mucosa, but this occurs largely in children under the age of 10 years. Where it is suspected, ^{99m}Tc-pertechnate scintigraphy is the appropriate imaging modality, although some have argued that laparotomy is the best first step.

Case 17.4

1. a, e
2. c

This patient has glycosuria, with a low serum potassium and urate, suggesting proximal renal tubule dysfunction. In keeping with this, there is a normal anion gap acidosis. In proximal RTA, the amount of bicarbonate that can be resorbed from the urine is lower than normal, hence the bicarbonate wasting and acidosis. However, as the total body bicarbonate falls, the concentration falls in the urine to the point where the tubules are once more able to resorb all the bicarbonate. At this equilibrium point, the urine once more appears acidified. Therefore, a urine pH below six in the face of a low serum bicarbonate helps distinguish proximal from distal RTA, where the urine pH is greater than six. Proximal RTA may present with myopathy or osteomalacia. The raised ESR and total protein make myeloma the likely underlying cause. Note that myeloma may also cause distal tubule dysfunction, manifest as a concentrating defect. Unless there is a pathological fracture, myelomatosis is silent on bone scintigraphy.

Other causes of proximal RTA include:

- Vitamin D deficiency
- Lead poisoning
- Old tetracycline
- Hyperparathyroidism

- Wilson's disease
- Cystinosis

Case 17.5

1. b, f

Hypertension with biochemistry that suggests a state of excess mineralocorticoids (hypokalaemic metabolic alkalosis) but with suppressed aldosterone may be caused by congenital adrenal hyperplasia in children (17-alpha-hydroxylase or 11-beta-ahydroxylase mutations), Liddle's syndrome or the syndrome of apparent mineralocorticoid excess. Liddle's syndrome is an autosomal dominant disorder due to an activating mutation in the amiloride-sensitive epithelial sodium channel. Apparent mineralocorticoid excess is due to inactivating mutations in 11-beta-hydroxysteroid dehydrogenase, the enzyme that protects mineralocorticoid receptors from activation by high levels of glucocorticoid (the same enzyme inhibited by liquorice). Almost all sufferers have stature below the third centile. Glucocorticoid-repressible hyperaldosteronism results from a genetic fusion, such that aldosterone synthase is under the control of the 11-beta-hydroxylase promoter and hence ACTH. Thus, levels of aldosterone are high and suppressed by dexamethasone. All these disorders are probably underdiagnosed and may be discriminated by urinary steroid profiles. Note that the common causes of 'resistant' hypertension in clinic are surreptitious alcohol consumption, non-compliance with medication and 'white-coat' hypertension.

Case 17.6

1. c, f
2. a

Botulinum toxin blocks acetylcholine action, resulting in autonomic paralysis and weakness, particularly of cranial nerves. Symptoms develop within 12–72 hours of ingestion. Many patients have no gastrointestinal symptoms. Home-preserved food is particularly incriminated (hence the vicar's wife), although infected wounds may provide an alternative entry route. Symptoms may be very mild and overlooked or may result in a descending paralysis with autonomic involvement. Some patients have only autonomic disturbance, with, for example, hypotension, paralytic ileus and urinary retention. Sensation is normal. The toxin can be detected in serum, urine or gastric contents. Treatment is with anti-toxin and penicillin to eradicate any remaining bacilli, in addition to any supportive therapy necessary.

Variants of Guillain–Barré syndrome form the main differential, e.g. Miller–Fischer syndrome (ophthalmoplegia, ataxia and areflexia) or polyneuritis cranialis (diffuse cranial nerve involvement) with autonomic involvement. Nerve conduction studies readily distinguish Guillain–Barré syndrome (slowed conduction if demyelinating, decreased-amplitude motor potentials in axonal form but with no potentiation with repetitive stimulation) from botulism (reduced-amplitude motor potentials on stimulation with increased potential on repetitive stimulation). Diphtheria can produce similar neurology, but here there is no history of a sore throat. Myasthenia gravis would not cause the autonomic symptoms (dry mouth, pupillary paralysis). Ingestion of atropine-containing substances, e.g. belladonna, affects only muscarinic receptors and would not result in a descending paralysis. Toxic fish or shellfish produce paralysis of more rapid onset. If presentation was abroad, then tick-bite paralysis, neurotoxic snake bite and paralytic rabies would enter the differential.

Case 17.7

1. d
2. c

A moderately elevated prolactin may be due to a non-prolactin-secreting tumour compressing the pituitary stalk and decreasing inhibitory dopamine reaching the pituitary. In this case, the evidence of impingement on all the other pituitary axes suggests the presence of a sizeable tumour, and the visual field evidence suggests that the chiasmal compression is from above, making craniopharyngioma the most likely diagnosis (although eccentric growth of a non-functioning pituitary adenoma or another tumour, such as a meningioma, are also possible). Note that hydrocortisone replacement will be necessary during surgery.

Most prolactinomas may be treated solely with dopamine agonists such as cabergoline, with striking remission in tumour bulk being achieved. The threshold for surgical intervention in these tumours is thus high, being confined mostly to the debulking of large tumours causing compression of surrounding structures and to those patients intolerant of medical therapy.

Case 17.8

1. a, c
2. d

Common causes for a raised PCV or haemoglobin are the patient consuming alcohol the night before or taking diuretics. Alternatively, the plasma volume may be lower than normal, from an endocrine disorder or for no apparent reason. To exclude this group with relative, stress or pseudopolycythaemia, plasma volume and red cell mass measurements are necessary (a raised urea/creatinine ratio might be given as a clue in the exam). If there is a true polycythaemia but the platelet and white cell counts are normal and there is no splenomegaly, then it is highly unlikely to be due to poly-cythaemia rubra vera. Secondary causes usually result from appropriate erythropoi-etin secretion, e.g. carbon monoxide and COAD. If the pO_2 is normal, then look for an erythropoietin-secreting tumour. Renal disease is most likely, so the first investi-gation should be urine dipstick and a renal ultrasound or IVP. In females, do a pelvic examination and ultrasound to exclude fibroids. Then consider a hepatoma or, par-ticularly in young patients, a cerebellar lesion. The clinical history and examination make most of the options in question 1 extremely unlikely.

Causes of apparent (relative/stress) polycythaemia include:

- Diuretics
- Alcohol
- Adrenal insufficiency

Causes of true polycythaemia include:

- Polycythaemia rubra vera
- Secondary (appropriate erythropoietin secretion):
  - COAD
  - Smoking
  - Cyanotic heart disease
  - Obesity
  - Hypoventilation
  - Abnormal haemoglobin
- Secondary (inappropriate erythropoietin secretion):
  - Renal tumours, cysts, transplants, hydronephrosis
  - Fibroids
  - Hepatoma
  - Phaeochromocytoma
  - Cerebellar haemangioblastoma
  - Cushing's syndrome

Case 17.9

1. d, h

This patient is phenotypically female but has scanty sexual hair (androgen-dependent) and is tall because her joints have not fused. Together with the high gonadotrophin levels, this suggests an androgen deficiency or androgen receptor defect. A raised testosterone leads to the diagnosis of androgen insensitivity syndrome (formerly tes-ticular feminization syndrome). The non-descended gonads are at high risk of malig-nant transformation, as has happened in this case (evidenced by the very high beta-HCG and right-sided pelvic mass, formerly a testis). If there were no signs of malignancy, then the appropriate investigation would be karyotype analysis followed by laparotomy to remove the gonads prior to malignant transformation.

There are four syndromes with variable androgen receptor resistance:

- Complete testicular feminization syndrome
- Incomplete testicular feminization syndrome (some virilization)
- Reifenstein syndrome (phenotypic males but virilization incomplete)
- Infertile male syndrome (small penis and testes, oligospermia)

Note that if secondary sexual characteristics develop in a patient with gonadal dysgenesis, then consider transformation to a gonadal tumour.

Case 17.10

1. b
2. d

Budd–Chiari syndrome may present with fulminant liver failure or insidious ascites but usually presents with subacute ascites and tender hepatomegaly. The caudate lobe may selectively enlarge and the hepatojugular reflex may be absent. Inferior vena caval thrombosis or compression is often present, resulting in dependent oedema. Liver function tests may be normal. Seventy-five per cent are associated with an underlying pro-thrombotic tendency. Ultrasound gets full marks, as this is the easiest way to confirm the diagnosis. An additional thrombogenic tendency should be sought in this patient, even though she already has one risk factor. Treatments include resection of any webs, porta caval shunts, anticoagulation and liver transplant. Veno-occlusive disease is a non-thrombotic hepatic venule narrowing that mimics Budd–Chiari syndrome.

Budd–Chiari syndrome associations include:

- Pregnancy and postpartum
- Contraceptive pill
- Paroxysmal nocturnal haemoglobinuria
- Myeloproliferative disorders
- Venous webs
- Chemotherapy
- Nephrotic syndrome
- Behçet's syndrome
- Inflammatory bowel disease
- Veno-occlusive disease (graft-versus-host disease, radiotherapy, chemotherapy, immunosuppressives, plant alkaloids)

Exam 18
■■■■■■■■

Case 18.1

1. d

The typical history of straining and vomiting resulting in either a mucosal tear (Mallory–Weiss tear) or complete rupture is absent here. The rupture is usually in the left lower third of the oesophagus. It results initially in severe retrosternal pain. Later, fluid and air tracks into the mediastinum and large volumes of gastric contents enter the pleural space, with attendant shock. The CXR often remains normal for the first few hours, although mediastinal air can be seen in this case around the aortic arch. The later clinical findings are those of a hydropneumothorax. Surgical drainage and repair is usually necessary. Time is of the essence on first presentation, with only a few hours before mediastinitis and shock supervene. Early surgical referral is key: the diagnosis of this commonly fatal condition is often made late. (N.B. Hamman's sign is the systolic 'crunch' of intrapericardial or intramediastinal air.)
    CXR features include:

- Hydropneumothorax
- Subcutaneous emphysema
- Mediastinal widening
- Mediastinal air–fluid levels
- Pneumomediastinum

Case 18.2

1. b
2. a, b

Palpable purpuric lesions were noted on his shins. Raynaud's phenomenon and lower-limb purpura and neuropathy suggest cryoglobulinaemia. Cryoglobulin quantification distinguishes three types. Underlying disease associations can then be sought. Here, the positive rheumatoid factor suggests type II or III. The negative results exclude many underlying causes. Fewer marks are given for the less likely remaining diagnoses.

A leukocytoclastic vasculitis is seen in virtually all patients. Other clinical features include leg ulcers, abdominal pain, and liver and renal disease. The association with hepatitis C infection is strong. This is commoner in France and the USA. Liver function tests may be normal or deranged only marginally and fluctuant. Hepatitis C may also be associated with Sjögren's syndrome. Blood has been screened for hepatitis B for much longer than for hepatitis C. Treatment is that of the underlying disease plus reduction of the cryocrit by plasmapheresis if necessary.

Case 18.3

1. b, c, d

Note intracranial pus may block CSF resorption and the resulting hydrocephalus coning. Note that neck stiffness without irritation of the lumbar theca (no pain on hip flexion) implies a potential medullary pressure cone rather than meningitis. An urgent repeat CT is now necessary, with surgical drainage of the pus and intravenous antibiotics.

Case 18.4

1. e

Sum the white cell differential to reveal the eosinophilia. The one-month history of mild abdominal symptoms suggests an underlying gut disorder rather than a simple surgical obstruction. This was preceded by respiratory symptoms as the worm migrated through the lungs. *Ascaris* is the largest human intestinal pathogen, measuring up to 40 cm in length. Diagnosis is often made when the patient presents an emergent worm from the anus, mouth or nose. Ectopic migration may result in appendiceal, common bile duct or pancreatic duct obstruction. Larvae may be seen in sputum or gastric washings, and eggs may be seen in stool. This patient should be treated with a nasogastric tube, intravenous fluids and nasogastric piperazine citrate. Laparotomy would be necessary if no improvement was seen.

Case 18.5

1. a, d, e

Sudden cardiac death in an athlete has been defined as non-traumatic and unexpected sudden cardiac arrest that occurs within six hours of a previously normal state of health. In athletes under the age of 35 years, congenital cardiovascular disease is usually responsible. Collapse typically occurs during or shortly after exercise, suggesting that intense physical exertion is a precipitating factor. Sudden cardiac death is about five times more common in men than in women. The incidence increases in those over 35 years of age, largely because of the increasing prevalence of atherosclerotic heart disease.

The causes of sudden cardiac death or cardiac arrest in otherwise healthy people are shown below, approximately in order of prevalence:

Most common	Less common	Rare
Hypertrophic cardiomyopathy (HCM)	Ruptured aortic aneurysm	Wolff–Parkinson–White syndrome
Idiopathic left ventricular hypertrophy (possibly atypical HCM)	Myocarditis	Long QT syndrome
Congenital coronary artery anomalies	Dilated cardiomyopathy	Mitral valve prolapse
	Brugada syndrome (depends on population studied – common in SE Asia)	Commotio cordis
	Arrhythmogenic right ventricular dysplasia	Drugs
	Aortic stenosis	Unknown/other
	Atherosclerotic coronary artery disease	

Wolff–Parkinson–White syndrome, or ventricular pre-excitation, is present in 0.15–0.20% of the population and predisposes an athlete to sudden cardiac death. Athletes may complain of palpitation, light-headedness or syncope. The ECG may show an initial slurred upstroke (delta wave), short PR interval and wide QRS complex. Sudden death results from the development of atrial fibrillation with rapid atrioventricular conduction via a bypass tract and subsequent ventricular fibrillation.

Brugada syndrome has emerged over the past 10 years and has been estimated to be responsible for 4–12% of all sudden deaths and approximately 20% of deaths in patients with structurally normal hearts. The incidence of the disease is in the order of five per 10 000 inhabitants and, apart from accidents, is the leading cause of death of men under the age of 50 in regions of the world where the inherited syndrome is endemic (mostly South-East Asia). A typical ECG finding consists of a right bundle branch block pattern and ST segment elevation in the right precordial leads. This pattern can be present permanently or intermittently. Recent data suggest that the Brugada-type ECG is more prevalent than the manifest Brugada syndrome. In this case, prophylactic implantation of an implantable cardioverter defibrillator to prevent sudden cardiac death would be appropriate.

Case 18.6

1. e

This woman almost certainly has familial hypocalciuric hypercalcaemia (FHH), although the conjunction of primary hyperparathyroidism and vitamin D deficiency (producing relative hypocalciuria) needs to be ruled out. FHH is an autosomal dominant disorder with 100% penetrance. It is caused by a mutation in the cellular calcium sensor, giving an abnormal set point for PTH secretion. Thus, raised serum calcium and low urine calcium levels are seen, with a normal PTH. The condition is benign and requires no intervention. Note, however, that offspring may develop severe hypercalcaemia with a markedly raised PTH in the neonatal period. A 'normal' PTH level may be seen in primary hyperparathyroidism. This, in fact, is inappropriate: in the face of raised serum calcium, PTH levels should be undetectable.

Case 18.7

1. a, f
2. b
3. a
4. d

Antidopaminergic drugs are contraindicated in parkinsonian patients. This includes metoclopramide, prochlorperazine, haloperidol, droperidol and chlorpromazine. The only anti-nausea agent that should be used in Parkinson's disease is domperidone. Nausea is common early on in treatment and often subsides with time. Protein competes with levodopa to cross the blood–brain barrier, so the effective concentration peak is blunted if taken with a meal, particularly a protein-heavy meal.

Controlled-release levodopa is best used at night to ensure a good night's sleep. Its long half-life makes dose–response management difficult during the day.

Dementia with Lewy bodies is increasingly recognized as a common cause of dementia and should be considered in any patient with a mix of cognitive problems and extrapyramidal signs. Visual hallucinations, fluctuating confusion and falls are common. Standard antipsychotics are contraindicated, so management involves lowering the dose of the antiparkinsonian medication (all of which increase the chance of confusion and hallucinations, although dopamine agonists more so than levodopa) and, increasingly, the use of anticholinesterases.

An age of 68 years is too old for Wilson's disease. Multiple-system atrophy is a parkinsonian syndrome in which patients also get autonomic and cerebellar degeneration.

Case 18.8

1. a

This case illustrates the fundamental importance of acidosis as opposed to hyperglycaemia per se in insulin deficiency. 'Normoglycaemic' DKA is unusual but well recognized (around 3% of patients with DKA have been reported with glucose <16 mmol/l and fewer than 1% with glucose <10 mmol/l in one large series). This patient has a high anion gap metabolic acidosis. Bedside glucose estimation can be wildly inaccurate, although this tends to be in the lower ranges (e.g. the patient in a hypoglycaemic coma but with an apparently normal finger-prick glucose of 4). However, in this case the laboratory blood glucose was also normal. Other causes of metabolic acidosis need to be excluded. The pathophysiology of normoglycaemic ketoacidosis is poorly understood, but it seems to occur in the context of fasting prior to insulin deficiency. The normal biochemistry of fasting includes low glucose, high fatty acids, and a high rate of lipolysis due to counter-regulatory hormones. Thus, when insulin is withdrawn, ketones from fatty acids rise particularly quickly in comparison to glucose. Thus 'normoglycaemic' DKA is not likely to represent a discrete syndrome. Treatment is with fluid and insulin replacement. Dextrose infusion is necessary to prevent hypoglycaemia and allow continued insulin infusion. Note that if no urine is available to dipstick for ketones, then plasma can be dipsticked easily with a reagent strip. Alternatively, direct determination of plasma ketone bodies may be possible.

Case 18.9

1. c
2. a, b

Cricoarytenoid joint rheumatoid effusion may cause hoarseness, but you would need then to invoke another mechanism for the ophthalmoplegia and explain why all of the other signs and symptoms of active rheumatoid had resolved. Grave's disease does not explain the lack of palatal movement, and if it were to affect the voice, then other signs of hypothyroidism would be expected. A high titre of anti-acetylcholine receptor antibody is diagnostic of myasthenia gravis and removes the need for a potentially dangerous Tensilon test. The EMG findings are technically difficult to obtain. Here, the temporal relationship to the commencement of penicillamine therapy makes a search for a thymoma less relevant. Penicillamine-induced myasthenia improves within months of stopping the drug.

Note: reflexes are normal or increased in myasthenia; if decreased, think ?Lambert–Eaton myasthenic syndrome.

Note: patients presenting with bulbar weakness or aspiration from a 'stroke' – think ?bulbar myasthenia.

Other side effects of penicillamine include:

- Pseudoxanthoma elasticum-like condition
- Blood dyscrasia
- Goodpasture's syndrome

- SLE
- Pemphigus
- Rheumatoid arthritis syndrome (when used for non-rheumatoid disease)

Case 18.10

1. Leukaemia-associated pseudohyperkalaemia, familial pseudohyperkalaemia

The commonest causes of a spuriously raised potassium are haemolysis of the sample, sampling from a drip arm, and delay in processing a sample (samples that have been standing around a long time before the red cells have been removed suffer leakage from the red cells). The latter usually occurs only after many hours, but with very high white cell counts cells may leak and cause hyperkalaemia even if the blood sample is unseparated for only minutes. Rapid centrifugation may (although not always) help to avoid this. In familial pseudohyperkalaemia, abnormal cation transport causes a leak of potassium across red cells when stored at room temperature for only two to six hours. The problem is avoided by storing the blood at 37 °C.

Exam 19

Case 19.1

1. c, d, i

The incubation period for tetanus is typically 7–10 days, but it ranges from 24 hours to two months. In mild cases, the only symptom may be mild stiffness of the masseters. Treatment is with human tetanus immunoglobulin, intravenous penicillin, and muscle relaxants, paralysis or ICU as necessary. Active immunization is also necessary. Tonsillar and dental abscesses can mimic the trismus of tetanus. More severe cases can be confused with meningism. Reflex spasms of the affected muscles may occur, causing tonic contractions and complicating the issue further. The CSF is normal, however, in tetanus. Cases with marked dysphagia and pharyngeal spasms may simulate rabies, hence the importance of obtaining a travel history. However, there is no stiffness between the spasms of rabies and no trismus. Hydrophobia does not occur in tetanus. Ecstasy may cause trismus, users moving their jaws to prevent contractures, as well as a neuroleptic malignant-like syndrome. The diarrhoea was leading you towards botulism, which causes weakness rather than spasm and enters the differential of acute Guillain–Barré syndrome. Strychnine poisoning can mimic tetanus and some illicit drugs are said to be cut with strychnine (although this is probably no longer true). However, an acute dystonic reaction is certainly a possibility. The list of drugs implicated is legion, and occasional cases are unrelated to any medication. Hysteria is a possible diagnosis in this case but would be a diagnosis of exclusion. The actual investigations done would depend on how the case developed after overnight observation. Rabies, for reference, is best confirmed early in the disease by immunofluorescence of viral antigen in the nerve branches of a skin biopsy.

Case 19.2

1. a
2. b

The downbeat nystagmus localizes to the foramen magnum. The low hairline suggests a developmental abnormality. The ataxia suggests cerebellar involvement. Klippel–Feil syndrome is probably due to abnormal somite segmentation during development and manifests as fused cervical vertebrae, often with underlying cervical cord abnormalities, such as mirror movements. Like platybasia and basilar invagination, it is associated with a syrinx. However, Chiari malformations are by far the commonest association, the ataxia in particular making this the most likely diagnosis.

Case 19.3

1. f
2. f
3. c

Although this presentation could be seen in Rocky Mountain spotted fever, the long incubation period, the lack of rash, the diathesis for severe infection (due to splenectomy) and the classical geographic location point towards babesiosis. This is confirmed by the finding of intra-erythrocytic protozoa on Giemsa-stained blood film (these appear rather falciparum-like, but they are not pigmented and they may be seen in pathognomonic tetrads). *Babesia* are some of the commonest bloodborne protozoa worldwide and a relatively common cause of human infections in the north-east USA. The usual organism is *B. microtia*, which may cause a prolonged low-level infection or, occasionally, a fulminant and life-threatening illness. Infection may also occur sporadically in Europe due to *B. divergens*, which is associated with cattle. This is a much more severe infection, with 40% mortality reported. As in malaria, splenectomy predisposes to life-threatening infection, with massive haemolysis and renal failure. Treatment may also be with atovaquone and azithromycin, and exchange transfusion may be necessary in severe cases. Co-infection with *Borrelia burgdorferi* or *Ehrlichia* species is not uncommon.

Malaria and tick-borne relapsing fever are found only at much more southerly latitudes.

Case 19.4

1. d

Pick the hard fact with a small differential diagnosis: bilateral carpal tunnel syndrome. Now cross-check this differential with that of the nephrotic syndrome: amyloidosis and diabetes are left. The (random) blood glucose is probably normal, therefore amyloidosis is the most likely unifying diagnosis. There is no history of chronic inflammation to suggest AA amyloidosis (unless there is an occult neoplasm), so a search must be made for an underlying blood dyscrasia causing AL amyloidosis. Investigation may include bone marrow biopsy, urine Bence–Jones protein, serum immunoglobulins/electrophoresis, renal biopsy and rectal biopsy. Hereditary systemic amyloidosis is rare and often leads to neuropathy. Most patients with amyloidosis have proteinuria. Another presentation might be postural hypotension (autonomic neuropathy) and proteinuria. Other features include enlargement of the tongue, thyroid or liver, purpura, and a restrictive pattern of heart failure (especially in AL amyloidosis). Carcinomas may be associated with membranous glomerulonephritis and also many different types of neuropathy, but bilateral carpal tunnel syndrome would be unusual. N.B. paraproteins may also lead to peripheral demyelination.

Case 19.5

1. c

Gordon's syndrome is an autosomal dominant disorder that presents in the second and third decades with hypertension, hyperkalaemia and sodium retention but a low serum aldosterone level. The volume expansion may be due to an abnormally large loop chloride resorption, but the full pathogenesis, in particular the reason for the low aldosterone in the face of hyperkalaemia, is unknown. It is also known as type II pseudohypoaldosteronism.

Type I pseudohypoaldosteronism is an autosomal recessive disorder of childhood manifest by aldosterone resistance. The features are those of hypoaldosteronism (hyperkalaemic metabolic acidosis with salt wasting), but with a high aldosterone level. It is thus quite different to type II pseudohypoaldosteronism.

Patients with tubulointerstitial disease may have tubular resistance to the effects of aldosterone. An equivalent situation is achieved pharmacologically with spironolactone. Here, renin–angiotensin–aldosterone levels will be normal or raised.

RTA type IV refers to a hyperkalaemic normal anion gap acidosis. It results from any cause of hypoaldosteronism. Aldosterone increases the amount of hydrogen ions secreted across the distal tubule. Patients do not retain salt and are thus hypertensive.

Case 19.6

1. c, h
2. e

The scintigram shown here shows negligible uptake of tracer by the thyroid gland. Hashimoto's disease classically refers to the goitrous form of autoimmune hypothyroidism, but autoimmune thyroiditis in fact covers a spectrum from goitre to atrophic thyroid glands, and from initial thyrotoxicosis to hypothyroidism. This presentation is most likely the so-called 'silent' form of autoimmune thyroiditis. Treatment is symptomatic. The disease may remit spontaneously, leading to temporary hypothyroidism before euthyroidism is re-established, but around 50% of patients remain hypothyroid. De Quervain's thyroiditis (subacute thyroiditis) often follows an upper respiratory tract infection. Follicular destruction leads to an initial release of thyroxine but also to absent uptake on scintigraphy. Pain, tenderness, fever, a much higher ESR and leuko-cytosis are typical. Most patients eventually become euthyroid. Ovarian teratomas may harbour thyroid tissue (struma ovarii), which may rarely lead to thyrotoxicosis with a presentation like this. Scintigraphy of the abdomen would reveal local uptake of tracer. Note that factitious thyroxine intake will also suppress the thyroid gland.

Case 19.7

1. f

The HCG beta subunit is very similar to LH. It may have an LH-like action in stimu-lating Leydig cells and thus testosterone production, and it can cross-react with some LH assays. Seminiferous tubule development is dependent on FSH, and therefore a case of precocious puberty with small testes might be due to an HCG-secreting tumour. In high quantities, HCG has TSH-like activity; thus, a goitre and hyperthyroidism may result, but with no eye signs. Common causes are teratomas, choriocarcinomas and pinealomas. These often co-secrete oestrogen, resulting in gynaecomastia or dysmenorrhoea. In this case, the loss of up-gaze is striking and points to the pineal region as part of Parinaud's syndrome (which includes loss of conjugate upward gaze with normal convergence, and is not to be confused with Parinaud's oculog-landular syndrome seen in cat-scratch disease).

Case 19.8

1. d
2. a, h

Gaucher's disease is the commonest lysosomal storage disease (carrier frequency around one in 18 in the Ashkenazi population). It should be suspected in patients with easy bruising, splenomegaly and bone pain. Other characteristic features of Gaucher's disease are pigmented areas on the forehead, hands and pretibial region and pingec-ulae. Acid phosphatase and ACE levels are markers of disease activity. Infection may lead to a dramatic worsening of the disease. Definitive treatment is with intra-venous purified or recombinant glucocerebrosidase fortnightly, although in a few severe cases bone marrow transplantation may offer cure at the expense of the mor-bidity and mortality of the procedure.

Case 19.9

1. c
2. b

This patient has had dactylitis and has a raised calcium, dilated cardiomyopathy and a negative tuberculin test. Sarcoidosis explains all these findings. Anergy in someone with likely TB exposure suggests either sarcoidosis or lymphoma (100 TU is a high concentration). TB usually affects the heart through the pericardium. Myocardial TB is rare and usually occurs in miliary TB. Five per cent of cases of sarcoidosis affect the heart, with dilated cardiomyopathy and conduction disturbances being common features. A ventricular aneurysm in the presence of a normal angiogram is highly suggestive of sarcoidosis.

Note that clinical examination of the chest in sarcoidosis is usually normal until the onset of fibrosis. Serum ACE is more useful in monitoring activity than in making the diagnosis. The hand X-ray in sarcoidosis may reveal cystic changes in bone.

Consider sarcoidosis in patients with:

- Any neurological or ophthalmological syndrome
- Unilateral paratracheal lymphadenopathy
- Hepatosplenomegaly
- Maculopapular or violaceous skin lesions
- Heart block, pericarditis or cardiomyopathy

Case 19.10

1. c, d
2. c

Consider PAN with any major organ disease plus hypertension. Kidneys, heart, skin and gastrointestinal tract are commonly affected, but many other organs may be involved: stroke, retinal aneurysms, mononeuritis multiplex, hepatitis, appendicitis, pancreatitis, etc. It is a disease of small and medium-sized arteries, unlike the very similar mPA, which is mostly a small-vessel disease. In addition, mPA may produce glomerulonephritis and pulmonary capillaritis (classic PAN does not affect the lungs and the renal disease tends to be ischaemic).

In many cases, the differential includes any disease that may cause a polyarteritis and thrombotic thrombocytopoenic purpura. There is no need to resort to angiography here, as tissue has already been obtained.

Exam 20

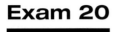

Case 20.1

1. b

The typical picture of Whipple's disease is a middle-aged man with a long history of seronegative small-joint arthritis followed by diarrhoea, fever, weight loss and lymphadenopathy. Other clinical features may include:

- Pigmentation
- Clubbing
- Pleurisy
- Pulmonary infiltrates
- Pericarditis
- Ascites
- Endocarditis
- Cardiac conduction defects
- Coronary arteritis
- Myopathy
- Eosinophilia
- Thrombocytosis

CNS involvement most typically causes a dementia-like illness, but a variety of focal deficits affecting all brain areas have been reported. Rarely, the CNS may be affected without any general manifestation. The Gram-positive PAS-positive actinomycete *Tropheryma whippeli* is seen in almost all patients on biopsy. The histological appearance can be mimicked by *Mycobaterium avium intracellulare* infection in HIV, but *M. avium intracellulare* is AFB-positive and *T. whippeli* is AFB-negative. Coeliac disease is rarely associated with dementia and myoclonus. Other enteropathic arthritides enter the differential, such as:

- Reiter's syndrome
- Familial Mediterranean fever (FMF)
- Inflammatory bowel disease
- PAN
- Behçet's disease

There were no painful skin nodules on the legs or abdominal or chest pains to suggest FMF, no renal involvement and a too chronic course to suggest PAN, no eye or mucocutaneous lesions to suggest Reiter's syndrome, and the dementia does not fit with inflammatory bowel disease. Vitamin deficiency may cause intellectual decline, particularly thiamine and nicotinic acid deficiency, but there is no other evidence of malnutrition. Limbic encephalitis is a paraneoplastic encephalitis, typically presenting with a subacute dementia and seizures.

Case 20.2

1. g

Osteoarthritic or spondylitic changes in the lumbar region in a patient with a congenitally narrow spinal canal may lead to compression of the caudal roots between the posterior surface of the vertebral body and the ligamentum flavum. Reflexes may disappear on exercise, and rarely disturbances of micturition and impotence may occur. Diagnosis is made by MRI. Treatment is surgical decompression. Rarer associations include Paget's disease and arachnoiditis following meningitis or myodil myelography.

Intraspinal tumours may be very indolent but are unlikely to cause such a clear relationship to exercise and no signs after three years. Spinal artery atherosclerosis could cause a similar syndrome, but there are no other atherosclerotic features and the aortogram was normal. Lumbar disc pain would be worse on flexing.

Case 20.3

1. a, j
2. d

Ileocaecal TB is a common cause of perforation and intestinal obstruction in some parts of the world, including Bangladesh and India, and has also been demonstrated to be relatively common in some immigrant populations in the UK. It is also increasingly common due to the HIV pandemic. Discrimination from Crohn's disease can be problematic, with more than one case report describing the institution of steroids for presumptive Crohn's leading to transitory improvement in wellbeing before rapid advancement of the intestinal disease and often perforation. Because of these diagnostic problems, good histological evidence is essential. This may come from peritoneal biopsy, laparotomy and biopsy, or ileoscopy and biopsy. In a Bangladeshi immigrant, Crohn's disease would be rarer than TB. Fever and splenomegaly are non-discriminatory. The barium follow-through findings are typical of TB. Ileocaecal TB may also present as massive rectal bleeding.

Case 20.4

1. f
2. d

Diffuse renal calcification is termed nephrocalcinosis, which is thus a morphological description rather than a diagnosis. The negative investigations exclude the majority of causes. Medullary sponge kidney is found in 0.5–1% of all IVPs and is usually sporadic, although autosomal dominance has been reported. It is characterized by multiple small dilations within the collecting system, within which calcium phosphate stones form, although hypercalciuria is no more common than in the general population. Providing infection or obstruction does not develop, renal function should remain normal. The IVP is characteristic, with dye filling the cysts before filling the pelvis, the dye surrounding the stones. Treatment is confined to recommending a high fluid intake (2–3 l/day) and avoiding instrumentation if possible.

Medullary cystic disease is an unrelated disorder in which cysts develop within non-functioning nephrons. Progressive renal failure ensues. There is no nephrocalcinosis. An IVP usually shows small, shrunken kidneys but does not outline the cysts. It is often familial, and postural hypotension from salt wasting is not uncommon.

Other causes of nephrocalcinosis include:

- Any cause of hypercalcaemia or hypercalciuria
- Hyperoxaluria
- Renal tubular acidosis
- Tuberculosis
- Chronic glomerulonephritis (cortical)

Case 20.5

1. a, e

This patient has chronic liver disease, which is most likely due to chronic alcohol abuse in the absence of other indications. He also has signs of haemolysis (recent shortness of breath, anaemia, spherocytosis, reticulocytosis and a high bilirubin) and hypertriglyceridaemia (lipaemia retinalis). The unifying diagnosis is Zieve's syndrome, in which red-cell osmotic fragility is increased after an alcohol binge (it is normally decreased in liver disease) in association with very pronounced hyperlipidaemia and alcoholic liver disease. PBC would not explain the haemolysis, so one would have to postulate an associated autoimmune haemolytic anaemia. PBC is also much commoner in women and typically presents with cholestatic features, e.g. scratch marks. Palmar erythema and spider naevi are comparatively uncommon, in contrast to alcoholic cirrhosis.

Note: alcohol is the commonest cause of a generalized increase in lipids.

Note: Wilson's disease may present with acute haemolysis. Evan's syndrome features autoimmune thrombocytopoenia and haemolytic anaemia.

Other possible presenting features of alcoholism include:

- Premature osteoporosis
- Cardiomyopathy
- Painful neuropathy
- Parotid enlargement
- Pseudo-Cushing's syndrome
- Via associated nutritional deficiencies

Case 20.6

1. a
2. a, b

Malabsorption plus a raised serum folate (from bacterial production) suggests bacterial overgrowth. Multiple fluid levels suggest bowel obstruction, multiple strictures from Crohn's disease or jejunal diverticulosis. There is nothing to suggest bowel obstruction or Crohn's disease, and therefore the most likely diagnosis is jejunal diverticulosis. Breath testing (2-h 50-g glucose hydrogen breath test) and jejunal aspirate and culture will confirm bacterial overgrowth, while imaging is necessary to uncover the cause. Here, a small-bowel meal would reveal jejunal diverticulosis, as shown below.

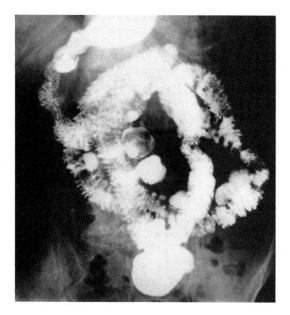

Causes of bacterial overgrowth include:

- Gastric hypochlorhydria (drugs, atrophy, surgery)
- Anatomical abnormalities (surgery, fistulae, diverticulae, strictures, adhesions)
- Abnormal motility (scleroderma, neuropathy, amyloid)
- Hypogammaglobulinaemia

Case 20.7

1. a, e, f
2. a, e

Protocols for diagnosing Cushing's syndrome vary from institution to institution, but the general principles are as follows:

1. Screen for hypercortisolism (e.g. three urinary free cortisols over 24 hours)
2. Confirm hypercortisolism (low-dose dexamethasone suppression test)
3. Rule out pseudo-Cushing's and then establish whether ACTH-dependent or not (circadian rhythm of ACTH and cortisol, CRH stimulation)
4. If ACTH-dependent, differentiate ectopic from pituitary (e.g. CRH test, BIPSS, high-dose dexamethasone suppression test)
5. Image the possible sites of the underlying hormone hypersecretion

Low-dose dexamethasone testing has a sensitivity of around 98% for hypercortisolism. Many centres now add CRH stimulation with ACTH measurement to the end of this. No ACTH response suggests pseudo-Cushing's (assuming the cortisol did not suppress), while a brisk ACTH response suggests that a corticotroph pituitary adenoma is most likely.

The distinction of ectopic ACTH from Cushing's disease is one of the more demanding aspects of diagnosis. In practice, no test is 100% sensitive and specific, so many algorithms combine tests. In expert hands, BIPPS is very reliable and may give useful lateralizing information prior to hypophysectomy. It carries a very small risk of severe complications, such as pontine infarcts.

Note that liver enzyme inducers such as phenytoin or rifampicin will accelerate dexamethasone metabolism and may result in a false-positive low-dose dexamethasone suppression result. Pseudo-Cushing's syndrome from severe depression or alcoholism may show loss of circadian rhythm. It will often suppress with low-dose dexamethasone, although in real life it may only suppress with high dose. Another discriminator is cortisol response to the insulin tolerance test: levels rise in depression but not in Cushing's syndrome.

Always consider MEN with Cushing's disease.

Note the rarities of Carney's syndrome (autosomal dominant), which consists of peripheral nerve and endocrine tumours, myxomas and spotty skin pigmentation, and McCune–Albright syndrome, which consists of fibrous dysplasia, 'coast-of-Maine' pigmentation, and gland hyperfunction (adrenal, thyroid, gonads, pituitary).

ACTH-dependent causes of Cushing's syndrome include:

- Pituitary adenoma (80%)
- Ectopic ACTH (20%), e.g. lung small-cell carcinoma, carcinoid, islet cell tumour, phaeochromocytoma, medullary carcinoma of the thyroid
- Ectopic CRF (rare)

Non-ACTH-dependent causes of Cushing's syndrome include:

- Exogenous glucocorticoid
- Adrenal adenoma (40–50%)
- Adrenal carcinoma (40–50%)
- Primary pigmented nodular adrenal disease (about 50% part of Carney complex)
- McCune–Albright syndrome
- Idiopathic macronodular adrenal disease (MAD)
- MAD due to ectopic/increased hormone receptors on adrenal cells

Case 20.8

1. h

This man has hypoglycaemia, a high anion gap acidosis, and coma. This is all suggestive of hepatic encephalopathy. The clues to haemochromatosis are the 'gout' (more likely pseudogout – characteristically in the second and third MCP joints) and diabetes. The pigmentation is disguised by his racial origin, although careful examination is likely to have revealed signs of chronic liver disease. Haemochromatosis is usually caused by homozygosity for the C282Y mutation in the hereditary haemochromatosis gene, but its penetrance is now thought to be rather low, although liver damage may be potentiated by concomitant alcohol abuse. Encephalopathy is a rather unusual presentation but has been described in the setting of a superadded insult such as sepsis, oral iron therapy, or the development of carcinoma, which is particularly common in haemochromatosis, developing in around 30% of untreated cirrhotic patients. The PT is the best monitor of liver function and is used to time transplantation. FFP should therefore be avoided if possible. The deranged clotting should be corrected, however, prior to lumbar puncture. As more liver is destroyed, liver enzyme levels may actually fall. Thus, these are not such good markers.

Other features of hepatocellular failure are uncontrolled bleeding and ascites. Treatment is supportive, with correction of electrolyte disturbance and hypoglycaemia, treatment of infection, and prevention of gastrointestinal bleeding. Intubation and paralysis with placement of an intracranial bolt to try to maintain the cerebral perfusion pressure (intracranial pressure minus mean arterial pressure) may be necessary while waiting for recovery or a liver transplant.

Causes of sub/fulminant hepatic failure to consider include:

- Viral hepatitis
- Halothane
- Paracetamol overdose
- Wilson's disease
- Acute fatty liver of pregnancy
- Autoimmune chronic active hepatitis (associated with anti-LKM antibodies)
- Solvents
- Amanita mushrooms
- Budd–Chiari syndrome
- Veno-occlusive disease (including post-irradiation or chemotherapy)
- Hypoxia (e.g. post-cardiac arrest)
- Sodium valproate
- Tetracycline
- Alcoholic hepatitis

Always consider other causes of coma in somebody with ?hepatic encephalopathy, namely Wernicke's encephalopathy, status epilepticus, subdural haematoma, hypoglycaemia, meningitis and intoxication.

Cases with secondary diabetes are common, such as:

- Some of arthritis, heart failure, diabetes, hypogonadism and liver disease – ?haemochromatosis
- Some of headache, sweating, diabetes and hypertension – ?acromegaly

Case 20.9

1. f, h
2. i

This patient is most likely to have MEN2A (medullary carcinoma of the thyroid, phaeochromocytoma and hyperparathyroidism). In this setting, phaeochromocytomas characteristically are benign and episodically secrete adrenaline, meaning that hypertension is often paroxysmal rather than sustained in the early stages, and beta-adrenergic symptoms predominate (fear, palpitation, tachycardia). The ECG shows only sinus tachycardia. Other features here are postural hypotension and evidence of haemoconcentration. Phaeochromocytomas per se may cause hypercalcaemia, but it is more likely due to be parathyroid hyperplasia in this case. The diarrhoea may be due to medullary thyroid carcinoma (MCT), seen in almost all cases. Catecholamine excess should be proven and controlled prior to surgery, and the *ret* proto-oncogene should be screened (also enabling predictive genetic testing when the mutation has been found). A careful search for MCT is essential. Beware the potential for radiographic contrast media to produce a hypertensive crisis. Surreptitious drug-taking should always be at the back of one's mind as a possible differential.

Case 20.10

1. d

The shunt occurs in the chamber before the step up or down in saturation. Therefore, here there is a VSD, pulmonary stenosis and a right-to-left shunt.

Subject index

The emphasis of this index is on disorders and differential diagnoses; individual symptoms have not been included unless essential, or unless discussed at length.

Page numbers in *italics* refer to the 'answer' section. vs denotes differential diagnosis.

Index of medical specialties